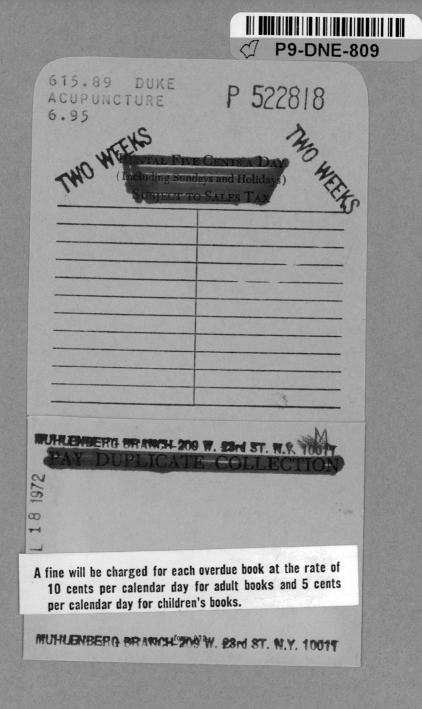

ACUPUNCTURE

ACUPUNCTURE

MARC DUKE

PYRAMID HOUSE
NEW YORK

Library of Congress Catalog Card Number: 70-189541

ISBN 0-515-09303-3

Printed in the United States of America.

PYRAMID HOUSE BOOKS

Published by Pyramid Communications, Inc.
Its trademarks, consisting of the word "Pyramid"
and the portrayal of a pyramid, are registered in
the United States Patent Office.

PYRAMID COMMUNICATIONS, INC.
919 Third Avenue, New York, N.Y. 10022

Distributed in Canada by
Pyramid Books of Canada
888 DuPont Street
Toronto, Ontario

FOR PAMELA

ACKNOWLEDGMENTS

Many people and organizations contributed to the making of this book. It is not possible to thank all of them here; the list is much too long. I would, however, like to mention a few that have been of particular assistance. Of the organizations, the American Medical Association, for their continuing advice; the Johns Hopkins Institute of the History of Medicine, which provided many of the sources used, and the staff of its Welch Medical Library, who offered their unqualified aid in my research. Of the individuals, Arthur W. Galston and Victor Sidel, who eagerly related their recent experiences in Communist China; Oscar Collier, whose belief in the project helped make it possible; John W.C. Fox, whose boldness in medicine will be singularly responsible for bringing about the use of acupuncture in the United States; and Pat Golbitz, without whose editorial guidance the book could not have been written.

Certain individuals have provided the support needed for me to successfully transform the immense Chinese experience in medicine into writing. Their help has been more personal than professional, but nonetheless essential. They are: Mrs. Harriet Myer, who transcended a great personal tragedy and continued to be a daily pillar of encouragement; H.F. Sunday, a silent, accepting, uncritical friend; Mr. and Mrs. M. Lavoie; and Mr. and Mrs. J. Goodman.

Finally, I must extend my gratitude, appreciation, and love to those people whose contribution goes beyond any measure, and who have accepted my trials as their own: my mother, my father and my two lovely sisters.

INTRODUCTION

"China was not discovered by Henry Kissinger nor acupuncture invented by James Reston", a Chinese physician and medical researcher friend of mine remarked recently when I asked him to translate a Chinese medical acupuncture article for me. As an American anesthesiologist I simply cannot afford to ignore the reports of remarkable progress made in my specialty in the People's Republic of China. Medical men and the public alike have been faced with the need to know about acupuncture anesthesia before even knowing that a branch of classical Chinese medicine called acupuncture existed. This book, written not by an American physician-acupuncturist (because as yet there are none), but by a concerned American Sinologist who believes that acupuncture offers much in both general medicine and non-chemical anesthesia, is a first.

A short time ago China became accessible to Americans after a lapse of more than two decades. What was the reaction to acupuncture anesthesia? Three patterns common to laymen and physicians emerged. The first was indifference. The second was skepticism and outright denial with suggestions of fraud, deception, or in some way political propaganda. The third and minority response ranged from the open-minded searching for more facts to the desperate grasping at anything that could possibly bring relief of pain or cure of diseases for which there is currently no hope.

Does acupuncture really work? In China, Japan,

the Soviet Union, Europe, and South America many patients and doctors are convinced that it does.

Marc Duke's book gives an account of the history, classical philosophy, and theory of medical acupuncture which has served Chinese acupuncturists for literally thousands of years. Tao, Yin, Yang, Points, Meridians, and the Five Elements provide an internally consistent explanation of acupuncture, but are generally unacceptable to Western trained physicians.

Here lies the problem for the unbiased investigation and use of acupuncture in the United States. In something so new and controversial, even favorable results based upon "unacceptable" theory tend to cause rejection of the entire method. Some parts of this book are bound to raise more than eyebrows; indeed there are portions with which I disagree.

Does acupuncture anesthesia work outside China? In October, 1971, a patient in Marseille, France, had a ganglion removed from the wrist, and in December of the same year a patient in Lausanne, Switzerland, had a cyst removed from the neck—both of these operations were performed under acupuncture anesthesia. I know personally the two physicians involved.

On December 8, 1971, two American anesthesiologists in New York volunteered to have acupuncture tried on them by a British physician-acupuncturist. A Chinese language text was used to locate the points used for appendectomy. First, each volunteer's abdomen was tested for normal sensation to pain by pin prick and pinching. After twenty minutes of constant needle stimulation of two points on the right leg, one volunteer reported a marked reduction to pin prick and pinch pain in the right lower quadrant of the abdomen. The two physicians were my wife, also an anesthesiologist, and myself.

The technique of pain control during surgery by acupuncture is of crucial importance to patients and doctors alike. At some future date when an American patient undergoes surgery with acupuncture anesthesia and experiences no pain the big question about acupuncture will be answered.

Pain is so real to all of us that it is hard to believe so much is as yet unknown about it. No single neurophysiological explanation accounts satisfactorily for all pain conditions; the ways in which some unusual techniques relieve or prevent pain are quite puzzling. Professor Ronald Melzack of McGill University has evidence that in the spinal cord and brain there is a sort of gate mechanism which can be "opened" allowing pain impulses to go to the conscious level or, under other circumstances "closed," preventing the feeling of pain. There are instances reported in Western medical literature in which stimulation applied to parts of the body far removed from the site of pain resulted in temporary or permanent relief of that pain. One was the observation that a chemical refrigerant spray applied to the shins stopped an artificially induced toothache for hours. Some of the acupuncture points used by modern Chinese acupuncturists to produce anesthesia are located in this area.

When a Chinese medical delegation visited McGill University in Montreal, Canada, in the Autumn of 1971, official films of surgery performed under acupuncture were shown and the Chinese surgeon and acupuncturist answered a multitude of questions relating to Chinese medicine and acupuncture. Dr. Melzack who some time ago proposed the gate control theory of pain, was in the audience. He was impressed with what he had seen and heard. Many apparently unrelated observations and experiments he and other psychologists and neurophysiologists knew about began to fall into place.

Much research still lies ahead in establishing a Western neurological basis for acupuncture. It may be

a long journey but the Chinese have taken innumer-
able steps in five millennia. This book represents a first,
large American step in calling the public's attention to
that new but ancient system of medicine.

J. W. C. Fox, M.D.
Assistant Professor of Anesthesiology
Downstate Medical Center, S.U.N.Y.
Brooklyn   January 1972

TABLE OF CONTENTS

ILLUSTRATIONS

CHAPTER I

THE STARTLING CURES

A thing is good only when it brings real benefit to the masses of people.
—MAO TSE-TUNG

AT THE Peking Hospital of Chinese Medicine, in 1966, physicians gathered 151 paraplegics who had been pronounced incurable by Western doctors. All had lost the power of movement from the waist down. The doctors began prodding their patients with long steel needles. Soon, some were able to wiggle their toes and feet, then bend their knees, and finally move their entire legs. They exercised for hours each day, rebuilding wasted muscles and gaining back the confidence lost in years of paralysis.

Thirty-six months after the acupuncture treatments started, 124 of the 151 patients were able to walk without the aid of another person.* China's doctors had accomplished the impossible, using a five-thousand-year-old medical technique.

Doctors trained in the traditional healing techniques —acupuncture, herb medicine, and massage—practice in every major hospital and clinic in China. The art of sticking sharp needles into the skin to cure illness and

---

* The cures are documented in French and Soviet medical journals.

1

disease today stands beside chemotherapy for cancer and open-heart surgery. In old China, acupuncture and herb remedies were the only methods used to cure illness. They were prescribed for every affliction known to man, from simple colds to malaria to smallpox. Acupuncture healed China's sick, whether they were peasants or emperors.

The emperors are gone now, and the peasants are comrades in a socialist state. Acupuncture is practiced daily in the villages that still dot China's landscape, although most are now called communes. The ancient healing art is performed in the same way it has been since the beginning of Chinese history, curing the same hundreds of illnesses it has always cured. But for the new China, there is also a new acupuncture, more revolutionary in the field of medicine than Maoist communism is in the arena of politics.

At the Hun Shan Hospital in Shanghai, a young man lies face down on an operating table. Chen Chien is twenty-four years old, a factory worker in the people's state. The operating theater is modern, ablaze with lights and filled with the finest electronic equipment available to medicine. Above the theater is a gallery filled with observers. Among them are James Reston and his wife. Reston, an editorial columnist and vice president of the *New York Times*, is one of the United States' most eminent journalists. He is in China at the invitation of the Communist government. It is the first time in twenty years that American reporters have penetrated mainland China.

Surgeons hover around Chen Chien. Chen has tuberculosis, an advanced case that will require removing his left lung and one rib. The surgeons deftly split open Chen's back, cut through the bone and muscle, sever and remove the lung and rib. Through the gaping hole, his right lung is visible, heaving and subsiding as it takes over the work of two lungs, bringing oxygen to his body and keeping the young man alive.

As the operation progresses, the people in the gallery hear an unbelievable conversation. Chen Chien, in the midst of one of the most difficult and serious operations known to medicine, has remarked that he is hungry. An attendant offers him some fruit, slices of orange grown in the South of China. He thanks the surgeons, eats the fruit, and answers a few questions they ask. Chen's voice is calm; there is no indication that he feels any pain.

The Restons are amazed, as they will later report to the American public over network television. Chen was conscious throughout the operation. He had been given neither oral nor intravenous anesthesia. One acupuncture needle, inserted in his right shoulder, deadened the pain in his entire body while the surgeons worked. For the few hours it took to remove his lung and rib, pain was a sensation unknown to Chen's brain. Still conscious, he was wheeled from the operating theater to his own room. The dangers and postoperative effects of general anesthetics had been completely avoided. Chen's body had to recuperate only from the surgery, not from the illness brought on by the potent drugs needed to put patients to sleep.

Hun Shan Hospital is the Chinese center for experimental brain surgery using acupuncture as the sole anesthetic. While he was there, Reston watched other operations. A forty-one-year-old oil field laborer had a small tumor removed from the occipital lobe of his brain as the journalist looked on. During the operation, the patient spoke frequently to his surgeon, Dr. Chiang Ta-chieh. Slim needles about three inches long were placed in his left hand and wrist as the only anesthetic. The operation was a success—and the patient felt no pain.

Chuan Liao, a fifty-four-year-old man, contracted

epilepsy because of a large tumor in the frontal lobe of his brain. Again, acupuncture was the anesthetic used to stop pain while a surgeon dug deep into the man's brain and cut away the abnormal growth. Chuan, too, spoke easily with his surgeon, and ate fruit during the operation.

Acupuncture needles subdued all pain in a thirteen-year-old girl who had a tumor removed from her face, with the *New York Times* columnist present once more. After the surgeon removed the tumor and stitched the incision he had made, the girl sat up on the operating table and walked back to her room unaided. Reston noticed that she was smiling.

The Western world's medical fraternity has been extremely skeptical of acupunctures' success as an anesthetic. If it works as James Reston saw it, acupuncture is easier, safer, and less expensive than any other form of anesthesia. Western doctors have pointed out that the operations Reston watched may have been staged, with some other anesthetic given to the patients before they entered the operating theater.

Their skepticism is unfounded. Acupuncture has been used as the only anesthetic in more than four hundred thousand operations in China since 1968. Photographs, films, and statistics have been released by the Chinese government to friendly nations. The technique has progressed far past the experimental stage, and James Reston is far from the only Western observer who has watched Chinese surgeons in action.

Dr. Arthur W. Galston, a Yale University professor of biology, travelled to China in the summer of 1971. At a Peking hospital Dr. Galston saw doctors remove a baseball-sized ovarian cyst from a middle-aged patient. Acupuncture was the anesthetic, this time in a different form. The needles were attached to a small generator. A tiny electric charge was sent through the woman's nervous system. It blocked all pain while surgeons removed the cyst and probed for other signs of disease. The woman examined the cyst after it was removed, while the doctors sutured the incision. She left the operating table as conscious as she had been when nurses placed her on it.

Dr. Galston and another biologist who travelled with him, Dr. Ethan Signer of the Massachusetts Institute of Technology, are not physicians. Galston specializes in plant physiology. Signer is an expert in the genetics of bacterial viruses. They viewed acupuncture as scientists, not doctors. When they asked, Chinese doctors told them that no scientific basis for acupuncture's effectiveness had been discovered, but that research workers were actively seeking an answer.

While Galston and Signer were in Peking, a woman in Wuhan made the question of a scientific basis for acupuncture seem frivolous. With a number of Canadian diplomats watching, a doctor performed delicate open-heart surgery. As he held a human heart in his hand, the wide-awake woman patient sipped orange juice. From her wrists and forearms, a number of stainless-steel needles glistened under the harsh lights. The Canadian observers could see that she was in no pain, even though acupuncture was the only anesthetic being used. As she left the operating room, the woman smiled up at the Canadians. The dangerous operation had been performed with unprecedented safety for the woman. The surgeon had been able to question her and accurately judge her physical condition. The woman's body had been free from the powerful chemicals used in general anesthesia and functioned during the operation as it normally would. She understood the procedure and approached the operation without much of the fear that is normal in people who face major surgery. She knew little, and cared less, about the scientific reason acupuncture works as an anesthetic.

Several thousand Chinese deaf-mutes, most of them

children, have felt the needles of acupuncture in recent years, not as an anesthetic, but as a cure for their deafness. They have been treated with needles as thin as a human hair for nerve deafness, a major cause of hearing loss among young people. In the West, nerve deafness is untreatable except by a delicate, rarely successful, operation. Surgeons must be specially trained to perform it, and the procedure is difficult and expensive. Hundreds of thousands of deaf-mutes live in the West; only a few score have regained their hearing through the operation. For China's deaf-mutes the situation is radically different.

At Shenyang commune in northeast Liaoning province, a People's Liberation Army (the military arm of the Communist government) health team sought a cure for deafness, using acupuncture, in 1968. They found that repeated insertions of the needles just behind the ear restored the function of damaged nerves. Deaf-mutes began to hear almost immediately—many for the first time in their lives. Combined with acupuncture in the patients' arms and legs, the cure proved permanent. The health team applied the treatment to 273 deaf-mute children in Liaoning province. In less than a year, 261 could hear perfectly and 252 were able to speak coherently and sing songs. *China Reconstructs*, a Communist Party propaganda magazine, described the achievement in October, 1969:

> "Deaf-mutes in the past were simply condemned as incurable by the bourgeois medical authorities. But a Shenyang P.L.A. medical team refused to accept this verdict. . . . The unit set out to alleviate the suffering of their class brothers by boldly applying the new acupuncture treatment. [The cured children] can speak and sing 'The East is Red.' No wonder they and their parents cheer 'Long, long life to Chairman Mao!' with tears in their eyes."

As with every Chinese success since the Cultural Revolution began, the new treatment for nerve deafness was attributed to the wisdom of Chairman Mao. *China Reconstructs* gave the official party line:

"By putting Mao Tse-tung Thought in command of their work, they created a new acupuncture treatment effective in quite a number of both common and frequently seen diseases."

Whether the new treatment resulted from "Mao Tse-tung Thought" or the five millennia of development in acupuncture, it did bring the sounds of life to thousands of deaf children. After the Shenyang discovery, health teams were trained to give the treatments and were dispatched to every corner of China. There are four schools for deaf-mutes in Peking. At one of them, Peking School Number Three, 238 pupils are enrolled. Since 1969 ninety percent of the students have regained all or part of their hearing after the acupuncture treatments. The students range in age from eight to twenty-two and are divided into small classes by ability. Peking's other deaf-mute institutes have slightly larger enrollments and equal records of success. Each month a few of the children leave them to enter regular schools, where they study the thought of Chairman Mao and become worthy comrades in the People's Republic.

The acupuncture treatments are not limited to children. In the city of Tientsin, a school and workshop for the deaf was established in 1959 during another of Mao's programs for China's betterment, the Great Leap Forward. Unemployed deaf-mute adults enrolled and studied sign language, then went to work making low-grade steel in primitive brick furnaces. The people were happy to be working again; all had been rejected by a society that found them useless because of their handicaps. Many of the 208 workers had families they were finally able to support. Their loyalty to the state and to Chairman Mao, if it soared then, became immeasurable when some of them were given the ability to hear. One of the men, a Mr. Kung, who heads the school's revolutionary committee, told a *New York Times* reporter what happened:

> "In 1968, the No. 626 propaganda team of the People's Liberation Army came to heal us. They did acupuncture on us, the new deep acupuncture that the medical team of the Army had perfected to cure deafness. Some of us had never spoken before. Some still cannot speak. But others, like me, now speak."

Of the 208 people at the school, one hundred now can hear. The rest continue receiving acupuncture, and all have hope. The percentage of people cured is not as high in Tientsin as it is among the children in Peking. Chinese doctors have found that acupuncture works best on young patients whose deafness was caused by childhood disease.

Acupuncturists are relieving another serious childhood problem with their needles: the crippling effects of infantile paralysis. Through acupuncture treatments given in the legs, Chinese children paralyzed by polio have been able to walk again, to join their friends in the daily marching and singing—most of which extols the great thought of Chairman Mao. The procedure was also developed at Shenyang commune in 1968. In the first six months after researchers discovered it, five thousand children were treated, again by medical teams dispatched throughout the countryside. Now, three times that number receive acupuncture each year. Exact figures have not been published, but Chinese periodicals consistently state that over half of the children regain complete or partial use of their legs during the treatment.

Other less astonishing but equally valuable uses of acupuncture have become commonplace in China— aside from the daily healing of simple illnesses. One needle, inserted a half-inch into the flesh between the thumb and index finger of the left hand, is all the anesthetic used by oral surgeons when pulling teeth or performing surgery. Acupuncture is widely used to cure arthritis and certain types of blindness. Doctors regularly employ the needles to stop convulsions and epileptic seizures. They achieve remarkable results treating emotional disorders, as Aldous Huxley noted after a trip to China. Huxley reported in the October 22, 1961, edition of the London *Observer* that acupuncturists, using the same methods described in ancient Chinese textbooks, were able to cure "certain kinds of depression and anxiety, for example, which disappear . . . as soon as the normal circulation of energy is restored. Results which several years on the analyst's couch have failed to produce may be obtained . . . by two or three pricks with a needle." Mental illness is not new to acupuncture. Chinese doctors treated it with needles as early as 2600 B.C., as they did every other ailment their patients contracted.

Treatment of common illnesses by acupuncture is far from obsolete in the new China, as James Reston found out on July 17, 1971. While touring Peking, Reston came down with a case of acute appendicitis. He was rushed to the Anti-Imperialist Hospital (formerly the Peking University Medical Center, endowed by John D. Rockefeller in the 1930's) where doctors told him his appendix must come out. Surgeons removed the organ under a spinal anesthetic, not acupuncture. Soon after the operation, Reston complained of stomach cramps. His pains were diagnosed as gastritis, a common complaint among patients who have just had their appendix removed. From across the hospital, an acupuncturist was called in for consultation. Complete with long black coat and skullcap, he examined the journalist and concurred with the other doctors' diagnoses. He asked Reston if he might use acupuncture to relieve the pain. Reston agreed. Three slim needles were twirled into his elbow and lower legs. After about twenty minutes, while the acupuncturist burned a Chinese herb, *ai yen* (leaves of mugwort), in front of Reston's stomach, the pain stopped.

Describing his experience, Reston said, "It's not at all painful. It tingles a bit, but that's about all." Reston's treatment drew headlines across the world; it was the first time an American had been treated by acupuncture in China and reported it. To the American public, acupuncture sounded like either a bizarre torture or a miraculous way of curing illnesses. It is neither. Acupuncture is a complete and effective system of medicine, as the Chinese are proving.

James Reston's doctors were not trying out an experimental technique when they called in an acupuncturist to treat him. Acupuncture is regularly prescribed in cases of appendicitis. In July, 1959, the Chung Shan Medical College in Canton published the results of clinical studies made on patients with acute appendicitis. Thirty-six cases were involved. The needles were used not just to relieve gastritis, but, except for a few herbs, as the only form of treatment. No surgery was necessary.

When they entered the hospital, all thirty-six patients had pain and tenderness in their lower abdomens, typical symptoms of acute appendicitis. Twenty-four had high body temperatures and abnormal white blood cell counts, also typical. Using acupuncture, doctors relieved the pain in seventy-seven percent of the patients. Blood counts returned to normal in seventy-five percent of the cases, and seventy-nine percent had normal temperatures after the needles were used. Every one of the patients was released within twenty-two days with his or her illness cured. The statistics include only those cases that responded within the first few days, although acupuncture eventually cured all thirty-six people. Unless it worked quickly, the doctors refused to consider the needling successful.

A number of famous people have turned to acupuncture for treatment of ailments Western medicine failed to cure. Prince Bernhard of the Netherlands, suffering from arthritis and bursitis of the shoulder, travelled to London in the summer of 1971 to visit a world-renowned acupuncturist, Dr. Yong Chai-hsiao. Two sessions relieved the pain—apparently for good, as the pain has not recurred. A year earlier, the prince received acupuncture from Dr. Yong Keng-no, a Chinese acupuncturist, in Singapore, for severe back pain. The treatment worked then also.

Premier Lon Nol of Cambodia suffered a serious stroke in 1970 and was airlifted to Honolulu, Hawaii, where the best American doctors available treated him. His recovery was only partial and when he returned to Cambodia's capitol, Phnom Penh, he called in an acupuncturist from Taiwan. The doctor treated the premier every day for a month, inserting needles up to three inches long in his muscles and joints. Lon Nol's recovery is now nearly complete.

These are the cases that reach the public's attention, cures of famous people who are considered worthy of mention in metropolitan newspapers. From the scarcity of these reported cases, the public might assume that acupuncture should be placed in a category with faith-healing, as a popular U.S. weekly newspaper supplement, *Parade,* saw fit to do. On September 26, 1971, *Parade* linked Prince Bernhard's acupuncture treatment to visits his wife, Queen Juliana, made to a faith-healer in Amsterdam. The supplement said of the royal pair, "The Royal Dutch Family is a most adventuresome

gung-ho group, apparently willing to try anything."
Anything, in this case, included acupuncture.

To the people of China, acupuncture is far from
"anything." Since the 1949 revolution, Western medical techniques have been available to the people. Uni-
versities train Western-style physicians and paramedi-
cal personnel, called "barefoot doctors," treat simple
ailments in communes and factories. Still, there are
550,000 traditional physicians in practice, as against
120,000 Western-style doctors—a ratio of almost five to
one. Prior to the Communist takeover in 1949, every
training institute for acupuncturists had been closed. By
1957, thirteen medical schools taught acupuncture and
herb medicine exclusively. Several hundred "secondary" schools were in operation, where health teams
learned to perform one type of treatment, such as that
used to cure nerve deafness. By 1967, twenty-one colleges of traditional medicine were open. At any given
time, ten thousand students are taking the six-year
course of study required to become a qualified acupuncturist. Throughout history acupuncturists learned
their art as apprentices to their fathers or to the village
physician. Sixty thousand traditional doctors are still
trained in this way at one time, providing a vast
resource of acupuncturists as older practitioners retire
or die.

In 1957 China had 144 hospitals where acupuncture
was practiced exclusively. More recent figures are not
available, but the number can safely be assumed to
have reached the two hundred mark. Also in 1957
there were 450 outpatient acupuncture clinics and fifty
thousand United Clinics (renamed Public Health Centers in 1958) where a Western-style doctor or nurse
works alongside traditional doctors. At the time of the
Communist revolution, approximately ten thousand
doctors trained in Western techniques were in practice,
with nearly four hundred thousand acupuncturists bear-

ing the major load of medical care for the people. They still do.

The Chinese people's lives are closely regulated by the state, but the people may choose to be treated by either traditional or Western medicine. Medical care is provided free by the state and the Communist Party sets doctors' salaries. If a patient needs major surgery, he may be asked to pay the cost of travel—which in China is very inexpensive—from his home to a large hospital. Otherwise he visits a local Public Health Center, where he sees the doctor of his choice, Western or traditional. The people's desires are clear from the overwhelmingly larger number of acupuncturists than Western-style doctors who practice. It has been argued that China has not had time to train enough modern physicians to replace the acupuncturists. In any country but China the argument would make sense. But Mao's government dictates exactly what each Chinese citizen will do with his or her life. Jobs are decided by the party, not personal preference. Western-style doctors are being trained at a slower rate than acupuncturists (when the apprentice system is taken into account, as it should be, since it produces qualified traditional physicians). Mao Tse-tung's government, damned as it has been until recently by the United States and other nations, may in at least one way be truly responsive to the desires of the people.

Acupuncturists treat their patients for hundreds of different ailments that cover the entire spectrum of illness and disease. Diabetes, high blood pressure, bronchitis, tuberculosis, cirrhosis of the liver, and schizophrenia are just a few of them. Between 1955 and 1959 the *China Medical Journal*, which has since ceased publication, gave cure rates for various illnesses treated by acupuncture. Chinese doctors claimed an average success rate of ninety percent in more than two hundred types of illness. As an example, acupuncturists cured 323 cases of tuberculosis, eighty-nine percent of those treated. But the figures are old and, because the state controls every publication in China, subject to questions about their credibility.

China is not the only nation where acupuncture is used. At the Hotel Dieu in Paris, one of the world's most respected hospitals, acupuncture consultations are held regularly, as they are at the Institution Nationale des Invalides, at Paris medical clinics, and in Lyon and other French cities. Doctors can specialize in acupuncture at French medical colleges; more than one thousand have already done so and are in private practice. Germany, Italy, Austria, England, Belgium, Brazil, Switzerland, Argentina, Japan, Taiwan, Thailand, Korea, the Soviet Union, and Canada also have professional acupuncturists. Doctors in most of these nations have done systematic research into the effectiveness of acupuncture. The results of this research unquestionably support the claims made by Chinese doctors. Every nation in the world that plays a role of any importance in the development of medicine has licensed acupuncturists and laboratories doing extensive research into the ancient art of healing, with one exception: the United States.

Not a single acupuncturist is licensed to practice in the United States, even though many qualified Chinese doctors live within the nation's borders. At the time of this writing, no hospital or laboratory in the United States has started to test acupuncture as an anesthetic or cure for illness. It is unlikely that any research will be started in the near future.

Why? The answer is difficult to accept: through a combination of ignorance and prejudice that in physicians is startling, the American medical establishment lags behind every nation in the world in its knowledge of Chinese medicine.

CHAPTER II

THE ACUPUNCTURE CONTROVERSY

Reading is learning, but applying is also learning, and the more important kind of learning at that.

—MAO TSE-TUNG

"I saw more of acupuncture than I know how to believe. As you stand there watching these procedures, your scientific brain says, 'My God, this can't be true.' But you're still standing there watching it. I'm still not sure how it works, but I have to believe there is some margin of truth in it."

The speaker is E. Gray Dimond, a few days after he returned from Communist China. He is not a journalist, or a biologist, or a diplomat. He is a licensed physician, chairman of the Health Sciences Department at the University of Missouri Medical School, and a world-renowned heart specialist. Dr. Dimond went to the People's Republic as a guest of the All-China Medical Association, along with Doctors Samuel Rosen, Victor Sidel, and Paul Dudley White. Rosen is one of the world's leading authorities on diseases of the ear. Sidel is a respected cardiologist. White, former personal physician to President Dwight D. Eisenhower, ranks as a patriarch of world medicine.

15

When the doctors left the United States for China in early autumn of 1971, the press rumored that they were being imported to treat Mao Tse-tung, who was supposedly on his deathbed. On his return, Dr. Dimond answered the rumor:

> "The Chinese have an excellent cadre of Western-trained physicians to care for their people. We went to China to visit with Chinese physicians about medicine. We did not see a single political figure, nor did we talk about politics."

Dr. Dimond saw a great many Chinese physicians, however, both acupuncturists and Western-style. He formed impressions about the state of medicine in China that reveal just how important acupuncture is, how widely it is used, and how much the people believe in it:

> "The Chinese aren't a bit out of date. Their best hospitals have everything ours have. I really had nothing medically to contribute to China. Their physicians know as much as I do. . . . Their equipment is as sophisticated as any equipment we have in the United States. . . . They are capable of performing any kind of open-heart surgery."

But the doctor saw that general medical care, the treatment of the masses of people for their everyday illnesses, was in the hands of China's acupuncturists:

> "The rural people of China have tremendous faith in their traditional doctors. Most of them have never seen a Western doctor."

The four eminent doctors were not marshalled through a propaganda tour of China's medical facilities, as cynical Western observers might expect. They were not led by the hand past exhibits of the country's most modern hospitals and clinics, or introduced to the most brilliant doctors available. Before leaving the United States Dr. Dimond compiled an itinerary which he gave to his Chinese guides. He was taken to every place he asked to visit, including seven hospitals in Canton and Peking and rural communes far outside the cities. He requested and was given permission to examine forty patients of his choice, which he did. He remarked on his return that the Chinese had kept a promise to him:

> "We were told when we entered the country that we could see anything we wanted to see and photograph anything we wanted to photograph."

Among the things Dr. Dimond wanted to see were operations using acupuncture as the only anesthetic. He watched ten of them. In one, the patient was a Chinese thoracic surgeon who had tuberculosis. Under Dimond's professional scrutiny, a needle one-and-one-half inches long was inserted into the patient's left arm. No other anesthetic was given. With the man on the operating table obviously awake and free of pain, the surgeons cut into his body and began removing the top half of his left lung. As Dr. Dimond remembered:

> "The patient's chest was wide open. I could see his heart beating, and all this time the man continued to talk to us cheerfully with total coherence. Halfway through the operation he said he was hungry so the doctors stopped working and gave him a can of fruit to eat."

Could the operations have been staged? One of Dr. Dimond's companions, Victor Sidel, thinks not. Dr. Sidel is Professor of Community Health at the Albert Einstein Medical College in New York and head of the Department of Social Medicine at Montefiore Hospital, also in New York. On October 18, 1971, the day after he returned from China, the acupuncture operations were still fresh in his mind. He believes the Chinese claims:

> "No question in my mind; I have no doubt that it relieves pain. These people [being operated upon] were wide awake. The method of pain relief was acupuncture."

Was it possible that the patients had been given another anesthetic outside the operating room? Dr. Sidel answered:

> "I would bet my reputation that those patients had no anesthesia other than acupuncture."

In another operation the doctors observed, a patient had a tumor removed from his throat. A single needle in the side of his neck deadened the pain of surgeons cutting open his throat, removing the tumor, and sewing up the incision. Dr. Dimond was impressed:

> "[The patient] sat up with a smile. He picked up the little red book of Chairman Mao's thoughts, waved it, and said, 'Long live Chairman Mao. Welcome to our American friends.' Then he buttoned up his pajama shirt, got off the operating table, and casually walked down the hallway to his room."*

What the American doctors saw amounts to only the tip of the acupuncture iceberg. In the rush of travel, as both Dr. Dimond and Dr. Sidel remarked, they were able to spend much too little time investigating Chinese medicine. Back in the United States, where most doc-

---

* Dr. Dimond's comments on acupuncture were recorded in the October 11, 1971, A.M.A. *NEWS*, a weekly newsletter circulated only to the A.M.A.'s members.

tors maintain an attitude of total ignorance and vague doubt about acupuncture, there would be little chance to use what knowledge they gained.

Doctors in the Soviet Union, on the other hand, have taken a long, deep look at acupuncture, and not only as an anesthetic. In 1956 three women physicists from the U.S.S.R. spent several months in China. The sole purpose of their visits was to study acupuncture. At that time the striking new uses of the technique in surgery and deafness and polio had yet to be discovered. The women observed acupuncture in its traditional, ancient application as a cure for all types of illness and disease.

They returned to the Soviet Union enthusiastic about the possibilities of acupuncture. The physicists so impressed their fellow scientists and the government that three institutes for the study of acupuncture—in Moscow, Leningrad, and Gorki—were established immediately. Extensive research was planned with a dual purpose. First, controlled studies of the effect of acupuncture on illness would be made. Second, a scientific basis for the effectiveness of the needles would be sought.

By 1959 the Soviet researchers were ready to announce some impressive findings. At the Gorki Medical Institute, Dr. U.G. Vogralik treated 250 patients with eleven different illnesses. All had been treated unsuccessfully with Western techniques. The illnesses included peptic ulcers, spastic colitis, bronchical asthma, hyperthyroidism, angina pectoris, erythraemia (abnormally high red blood cell count), severe facial spasms, and glaucoma. The patients were given acupuncture according to Chinese principles. No drugs were used.

At the Russian Acupuncture Conference, held in Gorki, Dr. Vogralik reported that seventy-eight percent of his patients were either cured or greatly improved. In every one of the illnesses, some of the patients' problems had responded to acupuncture. More than two-thirds of those with peptic ulcers were now free of them. Fifty-five percent of the patients suffering from glaucoma no longer had the disease. Forty of the forty-two people treated for angina pectoris, a heart disease, showed improvement. So it went down the entire list. In all, 195 people whose illnesses could not be helped by Western medicine had been helped by acupuncture.

A year later, in June, 1960, three other Soviet doctors astounded their colleagues at the Russian Acupuncture Conference in Gorki. Doctors L.J. Milman, E.D. Tikochinskaia, and N.P. Bobrova had been working in the acupuncture laboratory at the Bechterev Psychoneurological Institute in Leningrad. They had treated thirty-five men with a physical sexual problem—impotence—that Western medicine had been unable to cure. Again no drugs were used, only needles, as the long-established Chinese treatment for impotence dictated. The doctors reported that twenty-six of the thirty-five men, or seventy-four percent, were able to have normal sexual intercourse after being given acupuncture. After one-and-a-half years, twenty-four of the cured men were examined again. For all but three, the acupuncture needles had provided a permanent cure.

At the same conference, the other thrust of the Soviet research was discussed. Doctors had set out to find a scientific basis for acupuncture, one that went beyond the ancient Chinese explanation. The Chinese people believe that channels of energy, called "meridians," run through the body. In acupuncture, needles are inserted at specific points along the meridians. The channels and points are invisible and undetectable—or so they had been until the Soviet research.

Working together, three Russian doctors found that the acupuncture points could be detected by rubbing a sensitive stethoscope over the skin. The sounds heard at acupuncture points differed from those produced by other skin areas. After further work the doctors concluded that the skin at acupuncture points is less dense than at other spots on the body. Two other scientists, D.A. Galov and V.J. Piatigorski, found that the skin's temperature at the points is different than elsewhere. The Soviet researchers were making progress, but their investigation was far from complete (it still is not). But they had reached at least one conclusion: the acupuncture points do exist, exactly as the Chinese have claimed for five thousand years.

Doctors in other nations were not idle while the Soviets conducted their research. J.E.H. Niboyet of France wrote in his *Essai sur l'acupuncture chinoise pratique* that the electrocardiograms of patients treated for heart diseases by acupuncture showed a definite change, improving when the patient improved after sessions with the needles. German physicians announced that they were treating Parkinson's disease successfully with acupuncture—twelve years before the drug L-Dopa, the West's only reliable medicine against the illness, was discovered. Three Hungarian doctors proved in a complicated series of experiments that acupuncture cures numerous stomach ailments, even though the needles are inserted into patients' arms and legs. They published their findings in 1958 in *Deutsche Zeitschrift für Akupunktur,* a German magazine devoted entirely to acupuncture.

A Korean doctor, Professor Kim Bong-han of Pyongyang University, raised eyebrows in the medical world in 1963 when he announced that he had found definite proof of the existence of the meridians. Dr. Kim discovered that variations in the skin's electrical resistance could be traced along the paths of the channels and at acupuncture points. The paths corresponded almost exactly to drawings of the meridians in five-thousand-year-old Chinese textbooks. He also found that skin cells along the meridians differed in structure from most skin cells and that, at the acupuncture points, there were clusters of another unusual kind of cell. *Jen Min Chih*

Bao, mainland China's largest daily newspaper, praised Dr. Kim's work in a front-page editorial on December 13, 1963. The article, "Hailing the Profound Accomplishment of Korean Scientific Research," was accompanied by a full-page report on the doctor's work.

Meanwhile, French doctors, never to be outdone in medical research, sought conclusive proof of acupuncture's effectiveness. Over a period of five years, Dr. J. Mauries of Marseilles compiled statistics based on treatment by acupuncture of 625 patients. All came to him after Western doctors had failed to cure them. Each patient was examined by at least two doctors who concurred in the diagnosis. No drugs, not even Chinese herbs, were used to treat them: just needles. The following is a partial list of the illnesses Dr. Mauries treated:

> Lumbago, sciatica, facial neuralgia, cervical arthritis, gout, rheumatism in joints, tennis elbow, arthritis of the vertebra, arthritis of the knee, paralysis of the shoulder, spinal disc hernia, arthritis of the jaw, rheumatism after menopause, hay fever, asthma, emphysema, chronic bronchitis, cystitis, renal colic, tinnitis, sinusitis, laryngitis, tracheitis, deafness, menstrual difficulties, blood circulation disturbances, cardiac asthma, tachycardia, chronic diarrhoea, vomiting, gastralgia, constipation, epilepsy, Parkinson's Disease, diabetes, hyperthyroidism, Paget's Disease, eczema, dementia praecox, nervous hypertension, angina pectoris, excessive sleepiness, taenia, amyotrophia, excessive weight loss, seborrhea, anemia, obesity, vertigo, hiccoughs, insomnia, and psoriasis.

In all, Dr. Mauries treated 108 different illnesses. He succeeded in curing or improving the condition of eighty-four percent of the patients. Through acupuncture alone, 525 people were put back on the road to good health—after Western-style doctors gave up on them. Over one thousand acupuncturists practice in France. Many, if not most, of their patients come to them after first seeing other doctors. Their practices are large; acupuncture has become a leading specialty among French physicians.

A British doctor, Felix Mann, has done research comparable to that of Dr. Mauries. Using acupuncture, he has successfully treated over twelve hundred illnesses and diseases. In order to prove that a patient's psychology plays little or no role in whether acupuncture works, Dr. Mann has given treatments to men and women rendered completely unconscious by a general anesthetic. Even then, he found that the needles work, with results equal to those Dr. Mauries achieved. (Modern acupuncture needles are made of stainless steel. The material they are made of has no bearing on the treatment.)

France and Germany hold no monopoly over the use of acupuncture or research into its possibilities. Japanese doctors have found it effective against heart conditions and whiplash injuries. Czechoslovakian physicians use it to cure muscular trauma. Brazilian researchers are developing it into a form of hypnosis. In Italy, acupuncture specialists apply it to cardiac patients. Ukrainian pediatricians treat childhood diseases with needles. The British prescribe it for the mentally ill. Spanish doctors cure skin diseases with acupuncture alone. Rumanian dentists (and many others) rely on it in oral surgery and diseases of the mouth.

Between 1965 and 1970, medical journals in these nations and others printed 105 scholarly articles about acupuncture. It is considered to be a complete medical system capable of curing diseases that span the entire range of human ills. People in at least twelve of the world's most civilized countries can visit acupuncturists at any time they wish. Licensed professional acupuncturists treat patients daily in every major nation—

except the United States. Of all the articles written about China's ancient art of healing, only two have come from the United States. The May 12, 1962, *Journal of the American Medical Association* printed a nonscientific survey, nearly devoid of medical information, written by a historian. A similar article appeared in the *Journal* on December 6, 1971. The *Journal* is the American medical profession's accepted forum for serious, scientific articles on medical techniques. Other than in these two instances, the magazine has been silent on acupuncture—despite the research going on all over the world. A single example of what Chinese doctors have accomplished with acupuncture makes the tragedy of the situation apparent.

Using only acupuncture, Chinese physicians treat Type B encephalitis, a disease the West can do little to cure. When it strikes, Type B encephalitis often causes paralysis. Sometimes it kills. By 1953 Chinese acupuncturists had achieved a ninety-five percent cure rate of patients who caught it. The treatment is not available to Americans who contract Type B encephalitis. Most U.S. physicians are unaware that an effective cure for the disease exists. Since they rely upon the A.M.A. *Journal* for information, and it has chosen to remain silent, their ignorance is understandable—although, for people with Type B encephalitis, far from acceptable.

In 1971, when the cold front between the United States and the People's Republic of China began to melt, a trickle of communication started. Acupuncture began to make headlines in the American press. The attitude of part of the news media did little to help the reputation of Chinese medicine.

Life magazine, which is read by millions each week, printed a four-page story about acupuncture on August 13, 1971. It included a full-page picture of a man with dozens of needles stuck in his scalp and ears—a rarity in acupuncture. Above the article was a headline that said, "A visit to a friendly neighborhood sorcerer." It described the office and practice of an acupuncturist in Taipei, Taiwan. Rather than relate Dr. Wu Wei-ping's success or failure in treating the eighty patients who visit his clinic each day (he is Premier Lon Nol's doctor), the article dwelled on the "dingy decor" of the office and noted that it had "the practical atmosphere of a working magic shop." Most of the stories carried by other newspapers and periodicals ran in the same vein.

It is entirely possible that in Chiang Kai-shek's China acupuncture has the reputation of being sorcery. Generalissimo Chiang has never been fond of traditional Chinese medicine. When he held the reins in mainland China, before the 1949 revolution, Chiang attempted to pass a law making acupuncture illegal. At the time, fewer than five thousand Western-style physicians were available to treat the nation's half-billion people. Outlawing acupuncture and its more than four hundred thousand practitioners would have made medical care unavailable to nearly all China's people. The law never passed, because of strong public resistance.

With the flurry of publicity about acupuncture, opinions from United States physicians were inevitable. Virtually every doctor who voiced an opinion was skeptical about China's claims. None seemed to know about research done in other countries, but a few, such as Frank P. Smith, a New York neurosurgeon, had formed concrete views about it.

Dr. Smith, who heads the neurosurgical team at the University of Rochester Medical School, aired his feelings on a nationwide television news program in September 1971. "It's based on the Chinese calendar, not on medicine," he said. "I do not believe that acupuncture can cure deafness," was another of his comments. Concerning the rehabilitation of polio victims, Dr. Smith stated, "This alleged cure has no scientific basis." Neither, apparently, had Dr. Smith for forming his opinion, since no organized research on acupuncture has been done in the United States.

The battle, pro and con, raged on—and still does. As in every medical controversy, the American Medical Association has been brought into it. The A.M.A. is the largest organization of physicians in the United States. Sixty percent of the nation's doctors belong to it (the figure was once eighty percent, but the A.M.A. has fallen into disfavor among younger physicians). On acupuncture, the press has repeatedly quoted an unnamed "spokesman" as saying the A.M.A. has no opinion.

But the A.M.A. does have an opinion on every matter affecting health care in the United States, and a strong lobby in Washington to help make its opinions law. In the past, the Association's pronouncements have brought mountains of criticism down upon it, often wrongly. For example, when Dr. Andrew Ivy claimed to have found a miracle drug for cancer, Krebiozen, the A.M.A. turned thumbs down on the discovery. It said the drug had no value, that it was useless against cancer, and the research that followed proved the Association right. But before results of tests with Krebiozen were announced, the press, public, and thousands of physicians expressed their scorn for the A.M.A.'s judgment.

So the organization has become sensitive about giving out its opinions, whatever they may be. Acupuncture, however, is not a single drug. It is a complete medical system in use across the globe, in virtually every civilized nation but the United States. The A.M.A. could hardly afford not to speak its piece.

Piercing the "spokesman" curtain can be difficult, much like trying to find out who "informed sources on Capitol Hill" are. At the A.M.A. the man most often called "spokesman" is Frank Chappell, the association's science news editor. In a quiet voice Chappell informed

me of the A.M.A.'s stand on acupuncture. I quote him
with his knowledge and approval:

> "We don't understand it and we don't know any-
> thing about it. We know that it exists and that it
> has for a long time. But it hasn't come up so far
> in this part of the world. Remember, we are an
> association of doctors, not a research or licensing
> organization."

His next few remarks are noteworthy, coming from
someone who knows nothing about acupuncture. He
went on:

> "Acupuncture ranks with other Oriental folklore,
> but it can't be called medicine. There is a very
> heavy psychological element in it, possibly involv-
> ing self-hypnosis. Is there a scientific basis for it?
> It doesn't really matter. You know, if it helps you
> with the discomforts of an ailment you don't give
> a damn whether it's scientific or not."

Noting his statement that acupuncture does not classify as medicine, I asked him who might practice it in
the United States. He said:

> "It would be the practice of medicine, so it would
> have to be licensed. That is, it would have to be
> done by licensed physicians."

Frank Chappell's remarks reflect the opinions of the
A.M.A., as he assured me when I asked if he is their
official spokesman, and not his own. The A.M.A. wants
no one but a licensed physician to practice acupuncture. Its reasons are sound. Since acupuncture is not
taught at any medical college in the United States, it is
unlikely that many physicians will use it on their patients. It is hardly possible that the organization rep-
resenting over three hundred thousand American doctors is ignorant of a complete medical system, or the

research being done on acupuncture by twelve nations. Other reasons must exist for the lack of knowledge.

Most physicians are dedicated, hard-working men who earn their pay—and more. If acupuncture were to become common in the United States, doctors' incomes would fall. Surgeons and anesthesiologists would be the hardest hit if acupuncture replaced general anesthesia, as it might.

The huge amount of drugs American doctors prescribe would also fall. Fewer prescriptions would mean less money for drug manufacturers, another powerful lobby in Washington. Drug companies contribute huge sums of money to medical research. They are unlikely to support research into a medical system that is not founded on the use of drugs.

To the individual, acupuncture would mean far lower medical costs. Anesthesia, a doctor and assistant in the operating room, and expensive life-sign monitoring equipment comprise up to twenty percent of the cost of an operation. Acupuncture in place of chemical anesthetics would shorten hospital stays by up to thirty percent. Lower insurance rates might be added to the benefits.

Allowing only licensed physicians to practice acupuncture, as the A.M.A. suggests, would not prevent quacks from entering the profession. Anyone with a few needles—even the kind used for sewing—and a few charts of the proper points can, if he is foolish enough, try it. Acupuncture takes six years to learn completely, and sometimes longer. Few American physicians can spend that much time, on top of their already lengthy training, studying a new medical technique.

The American public need not wait until licensed physicians take up acupuncture. A few qualified acupuncturists live in the United States, but they are difficult to find and all refuse to admit that they practice the art, even on their families. Most will not even discuss the subject.

One who will is Ting Ching-yuen, a resident of New York City. Dr. Ting (*Mr.* Ting to the A.M.A.) is in his late forties. Born in Shanghai, China, he fled in 1948 when it became apparent that Mao Tse-tung would gain control of the mainland. He had just completed the six-year acupuncture course at the Shanghai School of Chinese Medicine. Dr. Ting was particularly proud to enter the medical profession. His great-grandfather founded the Shanghai school, and both his grandfather and father had served as its president. But history kept him from following in his father's footsteps, and he set up practice in Hong Kong instead. From there he went to Taiwan, Thailand, and Japan. At the University of Tokyo, he picked up an advanced degree in Chinese medicine, graduating at the top of his class after the two-year course.

Glowing reports about opportunity and freedom drew Dr. Ting to the United States. So he moved to New York, where his dreams were dashed. No license to practice acupuncture could be had, and after more than ten years in the United States, Dr. Ting, who may very well be one of the best qualified acupuncturists in the world, runs an herb shop in New York's Chinatown and is part-owner of a Chinese restaurant on Fifth Avenue. His years of training and his knowledge, which might be used to cure the sick or teach others the art of acupuncture, stand idle. In back of his herb store Dr. Ting maintains a small office, which is usually darkened, in the hope that he will someday be allowed to practice medicine again.

Like every other Chinese acupuncturist in the United States, Dr. Ting refuses to admit, even to close friends, that he still applies the needles. He is extremely fearful of being charged with practicing medicine without a license:

"There is nobody practicing it here. It is not legal. I practiced in China, Japan, Hong Kong, Thailand, and other countries. I have a license to practice in the Republic of China, but here I have no license. I cannot do it."

Dr. Ting believes that acupuncture has a place in United States medicine:

"I think now the people have no confidence in acupuncture. They know little about it. If the patients have confidence, acupuncture will work. It is medicine, and better than some American medicine. Acupuncture is five thousand years old. My grandfather and father practiced it with success. But now I can not. There are maybe fifty [doctors] in New York who have licenses from China. It should be available to American people."

Until the American medical establishment drops its pose of ignorance about acupuncture, Dr. Ting is not likely to find American patients appearing at his office.

Dr. Ting has not yet locked horns with the United States medical fraternity, but another man has. Reuben B. Amber holds a doctorate in traditional medicine from a school on Formosa. His teacher was Dr. Wu Wei-ping, the most eminent Taiwanese acupuncturist, Amber began his career as a psychologist, but turned to acupuncture after he heard of its ability to cure mental illness. Now he practices the ancient art openly in New York City, treating every kind of illness patients bring to him.

In 1965 Dr. Amber asked the New York State Department of Education, which controls physicians' licenses, to issue him a permit for the practice of acupuncture. The department refused, and also refused to rule on whether a license was needed at all. He went to the New York State attorney general's office and requested an opinion that would either allow the education department to recognize foreign acupuncture degrees, or prohibit it. Despite repeated requests, the attorney general has refused to consider the question.

Dr. Amber has only one recourse. At great expense to himself, and in the face of a possible fine and jail sentence, he must prepare a legal test case, which would force the courts to rule on the problem. Meanwhile, should the State of New York and the A.M.A. decide that acupuncture is medicine, he can be charged for practicing without a license. The A.M.A. does not want to make that decision. On the one hand it would be admitting that acupuncture is medically worthwhile. On the other, it would allow only licensed physicians to practice it legally. Unless the issue is resolved by the courts, acupuncture will remain unavailable to the people of the United States for many years to come.

With all the research that has been done in China and other nations, there is still no scientific answer for why acupuncture cures illness and disease. More investigation is needed, and if it is not done in the United States, which has the finest scientists and research facilities, it will surely be done elsewhere. But there is an explanation for acupuncture; the art of curing illness by piercing the body with needles can be understood. The answer is buried in the culture of China, the oldest continuing civilization on earth. It is hidden behind the Great Wall and the Bamboo Curtain, in Chinese proverbs and Mao Tse-tung's thoughts, and in China's unique writing, philosophy, and art. There the reason why eight hundred million people prefer acupuncture to Western medicine can be found.

Acupuncture has been called many things by people in the West: sorcery, black magic, faith-healing, miraculous. The ancient Chinese name for it is *tai chien tseng,* to "insert a golden needle."

CHAPTER III

MEDICINE IN ANCIENT CHINA

All things come from Heaven; man comes from his ancestors.

—Chinese proverb

EMPEROR I Tsung of the Tang dynasty sat brooding at his daughter's bedside. The young princess, renowned for her beauty throughout China, breathed heavily beneath the sheer silk curtains that kept her from her father's view. Waves of fever swept over her as she tossed and moaned in the grip of a severe illness. Attendants moved lightly about the room, not wishing— or daring—to disturb the supreme ruler of China while he contemplated his daughter's misfortune.

The emperor's daughter had been ill for many days. Potions prepared by the court physicians had done little good, and invocations to the imperial ancestors had, so far, gone unanswered. Emperor I Tsung was both displeased and worried. Abruptly he stood and rushed from the room, dictating orders to his ministers as the doors of his daughter's apartments closed behind him.

From the far corners of the empire I Tsung called together the finest physicians in China. His daughter, he told them, was his most prized possession. He implored and commanded them to cure her. One by one they treated her, some using acupuncture, some employing herb remedies. And one by one they failed to heal the emperor's daughter. Within hours after the last physician left her bedside, the young princess drew her last breath and died.

When his daughter's death was reported to the emperor, the wise men of medicine, China's most eminent doctors, were gathered before the Son of Heaven. In a bitter rage Emperor I Tsung ordered them all executed. The next morning, under a brilliant Chinese sun, the twenty best physicians in all of China were beheaded.

Emperor I Tsung reigned from 860 to 874 A.D., when Chinese medicine was already far advanced. In a calm moment he may have regretted slaughtering the cream of China's medical corps, but history records no remorse on his part. Like most of China's rulers, I Tsung had a huge respect for Chinese doctors and knew the stories of China's legendary emperors, who created the arts of acupuncture and herb medicine. He also knew of the great physicians of the past and perhaps wished, as life seeped from his beautiful daughter's body, that he had one of them around to treat her. Perhaps he even thought of the great Hua T'o, another Chinese physician who lost his life to a ruler's whim, but this time for being right.

Hua T'o was born in the administrative district of Po, in the province of Anhwei, sometime between 140 and 150 A.D. He became the greatest surgeon, and one of the most innovative physicians, in the history of Chinese medicine.

Hua T'o discovered early in his career that a mixture of hemp and strong wine would render his patients unconscious and oblivious to pain. He could then perform difficult and lengthy operations, such as the removal of brain tumors, without killing his patients, a noteworthy step in the practice of medicine. Hua T'o called his medication *ma fei san* and through its use became the first known doctor to perform surgery under general anesthetic. He used his potion in many operations, two of which insured Hua T'o a lasting place in Chinese literature and medical lore.

Kuan Yun Chang, the great warrior general, was wounded in the arm by a poisoned arrow during one of his battles. Kuan was a brave and chivalrous general who performed heroic deeds in behalf of the common people and peasants in distress. China's most famous historical novel, *The Three Kingdoms,* tells his story and that of the physician who saved him from death.

When Kuan Yun Chang came to Hua T'o with his wound, the surgeon decided to operate and suggested that the warrior take *ma fei san* to prevent pain. General Kuan refused, preferring to endure great pain rather than suffer the indignity of being thought a weakling. While Hua T'o dug into the wound with his knife, cleaning the poisoned flesh all the way to the bone, the warrior distracted himself with a game of Chinese chess (which is different from Western chess and is called the Game of Go in English). The brave warrior never flinched, as the many paintings depicting the operation show.

Kuan Yun Chang returned to his wars alongside Liu Pei and Chang Fei, two equally courageous soldiers he was bound to by blood-brotherhood. Seeing him return to battle, his arm fully healed and functioning a few days after being hit by a poisoned arrow, Kuan's arch-enemy, Ts'ao Ts'ao, wondered at the ability of his foe's physician. Ts'ao Ts'ao reigned over all of Northern China; the nation was divided into three parts at the time.

When Ts'ao Ts'ao became bothered by painful headaches, he remembered Kuan's miraculous recovery and decided to consult Hua T'o. Ts'ao Ts'ao appeared unannounced at Hua T'o's home and beseeched the doctor to treat him. The eminent surgeon examined the warrior for a long while. He gravely informed Ts'ao

Ts'ao that he had a brain tumor, requiring a serious operation. Hua T'o offered to perform it. But Ts'ao Ts'ao feared that Hua T'o's diagnosis might be a plot to assassinate him. He allowed the surgeon only to perform acupuncture that would relieve the pain. The acupuncture succeeded, and the delighted but ruthless ruler of the North attempted to keep the surgeon with him to treat his men when they were injured in battle.

But Hua T'o outsmarted the "usurper king," as Ts'ao Ts'ao was called, and one night escaped to the mountains in Honan province. A band of warriors was sent to search for him. They easily captured Hua T'o, who was by then about sixty years old, and returned him to the enraged general. Ts'ao Ts'ao imprisoned the surgeon and, when he refused to cooperate, ordered him killed. In the year 208 Hua T'o lost his head on the chopping block, as the twenty doctors who treated Emperor I Tsung's daughter would six centuries later.

As the years passed, Ts'ao Ts'ao had reason to regret his execution of the famous surgeon. The warrior king's headaches returned, this time coming more frequently and bringing intolerable pain. Eventually Ts'ao Ts'ao succumbed to them and died, not on the battlefield in a glorious exhibition of bravery, but as a man broken by disease. Autopsies were not performed in China at the time, but judging from the account of his death that survives, he suffered either from a brain tumor or another similar disease. It is almost possible to see the wise, aged Hua T'o stroking his grey beard and smiling ever so slightly as the departed Ts'ao Ts'ao entered the world of ancestral spirits. Hua T'o might even—although he did not—have created a proverb to cover the situation. It would have said, "Do not lose your head when you should keep it; do not keep your head when it is better to lose it."

Hua To's fame did not come only from his treatment of the two warrior generals; he was by far the finest surgeon in China prior to the twentieth century. Among the operations attributed to him are amputations, graftings of severed limbs, intestinal resections, and deliveries of stillborn children. In one of his obstetrical cases, Hua T'o diagnosed the death of a twin because of internal bleeding caused by the first twin's birth. The mother was in extreme pain, and Hua T'o knew that the use of *ma fei san* might be dangerous. So he neutralized all pain in the woman's body by acupuncture and delivered the stillborn second baby. The mother recovered without incident. Even in today's sterile operating theaters this type of operation can present serious problems for the best surgeons using the most advanced equipment and techniques. Seventeen hundred years ago Hua T'o relied only on his skill and knowledge and on acupuncture.

Hua T'o wrote under the name Yuan Hua, recording nearly every operation he performed. But his writings did not survive his encounter with Ts'ao Ts'ao— through no fault of the physician's. When he was about to lose his head, Hua T'o tried to entrust his written records to his jailer, who feared Ts'ao Ts'ao's wrath too much to take them. So, legend has it, Hua T'o gave them to his wife. Unaware of their importance, she burned them in the kitchen stove along with other belongings of the eminent doctor.

Fortunately for Chinese medicine, Hua T'o had a number of students, among them the famous pharmacologist Wu P'u, and reports on at least some of his work survived. In the eighteenth century Sun Sing-yen, a calligrapher, compiled what was known of Hua T'o's work into the *Hua-shih Chung-tsang ching*. The book is divided into three sections dealing, respectively, with medical theory, diseases, and diagnosis, and treatments and prescriptions. The work's fifty chapters contain some brilliant and far-sighted deductions about illness and medication, and show Hua T's's interest and influence in many branches of medicine.

Hua T'o originated hydrotherapy treatment and medicinal baths, both widely used in China today. Drawing on the knowledge gained from his many surgical operations, he compiled and published the *Nei Chao T'u,* charts showing the internal anatomy of the human body which are very accurate and are still widely accepted.

The surgeon made another valuable contribution to the Chinese healing arts. He believed that along with other forms of preventive medicine, physical exercise of certain types could aid man in keeping his body healthy. Hua T'o expressed his belief this way:

> "The human body needs to work; when it is in motion the food is digested, and the blood circulates in the arteries in all directions. Thus it is that the immortals of ancient days, while performing the inhalation process, and passing the time as dormant bears, looking around as owls, twitching and stretching their limbs and loins, and moving their navel gates and their joints, hindered the advance of old age. I have an art called the sport of the five animals: a tiger, a stag, a bear, a monkey, and a bird, by which illness can be cured and which is good for the movements of the feet, when they accompany the inhaling process. Whenever you feel unwell, stand up and perform the movements of one of these five animals. When you feel comfortable and in a perspiration, put rice powder on your body and you will have an appetite."

Hua T'o's belief in physical exercise and proper breathing techniques started an entire system of physical culture still popular in China and sometimes prescribed by doctors. Along with his other ingenious medical inventions, the surgeon developed the use of sutures inside the human body and pioneered in the use of ointments and antiseptics. As an acupuncturist he showed the way to many who would follow in his path. He was extremely skillful in employing the nine needles of acupuncture, rarely needing more than one or two to cure any illness. He set a standard that acupuncturists have followed ever since: the fewer needles, the better.

Hua T'o became so revered in the history of Chinese medicine that the people erected statues and pagodas to him throughout China. Prior to the Communist revolution his birthday was nationally celebrated on the twenty-eighth day of the fourth month. At his birthplace in Anhwei province, a temple stands in memory of him and his great medical ability. He has been celebrated for fifteen centuries as China's god of surgery.

The doctor from Anhwei and the twenty in Emperor I Tsung's reign are not the only Chinese physicians who have lost their lives because of their profession. Another doctor sacrificed his life to cure an emperor, and knew in advance that he would.

Dr. Wen Chi was the most famous physician of his time, credited with miraculous cures and superior skill in acupuncture. Had he stayed with his needles, he might have lived to a respectable old age. But he turned to psychiatry, and his knowledge cost him his life.

One morning the emperor of China, whose name has been lost in the many retellings of his story, awoke in a deep melancholy. Efforts to cheer him up proved fruitless and he slipped deeper and deeper into depression. He showed no interest in the affairs of state; reports from his ministers were met with a blank stare and silence. Neither the prince his son nor the empress his wife was able to break his mood. He was unable to eat, even when fed by his attendants with a spoon. Weeks of rest produced no change, and the royal family became worried that the emperor's behavior was caused by a serious illness, not some imperial whim. As the king became more and more remote from the world around him, his son feared that he would soon die and decided to call in the famous Dr. Wen.

Wen Chi hurried to the palace and examined China's supreme ruler thoroughly. He took the emperor's pulse, using the classic diagnostic method, observed his tongue and face, and listened to his intermittent moans, the only sounds he would make. Finally he stepped back from the emperor and called in the prince and the queen.

He told them that the emperor was suffering from a terrible emotional depression and nothing else. He said that only being thrown into a terrible rage would cure him. Wen Chi knew that the emperor, a normally benevolent man, was likely to do anything when aroused to anger. He explained to the royal family that to treat the monarch would very likely cost him, the doctor, his life. Wen Chi bordered on refusing to treat the emperor.

But the prince and the empress begged Wen Chi to do everything he could for the sick king. They promised that no harm would befall the physician under any circumstances. Dr. Wen agreed to put the emperor's life before self, and told the king that he would return the next day at the same hour. The emperor gave no sign that he heard Wen Chi speak, but the doctor assured the royal family that the emperor was aware of the next day's appointment.

The following day servants prepared the emperor for Wen Chi's visit. The appointed time came and passed, but the doctor did not appear. Hours went by, the prince and empress paced the floor in impatience, but the noted physician never entered. The royal family began to wonder if fear had overcome Wen Chi's desire to heal the emperor.

Another day passed, and another, but Wen Chi still did not come to the palace. A slight change in the king's condition became apparent. No longer did he moan. His face lost some of its blankness. Still he would not speak or acknowledge the presence of others.

On the fourth day after Wen Chi's first visit, the doctor appeared at the palace gates. He strode through the halls and rushed to the emperor's bedroom without removing his shoes as custom and respect demanded. Ignoring the royal family, ministers, attendants, and servants, Wen Chi burst into the room and began questioning the ruler in a mocking manner. When he received no answers, the doctor stamped his muddy shoes on the silk bedcovers and screamed insults at the emperor. The prince and the empress stood gaping at the spectacle of a mere doctor hurling abuse at the most powerful man in China.

Soon the emperor began to tremble. He leaped from his bed and ordered his ministers to seize the physician. He commanded that Wen Chi be immediately thrown into a vat of boiling oil. As though he had never been ill, the king ordered a huge meal, declaring himself famished, while the prince and empress beseeched him to lift his execution order. They attempted to explain why Dr. Wen had acted so brazenly toward the emperor. But their words did no good, and the royal hangman dragged Wen Chi away to be thrown into a caldron of steaming oil.

So strong was Wen Chi's will to live that he endured the torture for three complete days. Finally, he told the emperor's hangman that only if a cover were put on the caldron would he die. The emperor, still not heeding his family's pleas, ordered the vat closed, and Wen Chi's life and medical career ended.

Although Wen Chi's tale has little basis in factual evidence, and may entirely be the work of ancient storytellers, it illustrates two principles that Chinese doctors have always followed. First, the mind and the body are not separate entities to be treated apart from each other. Man's physical and mental problems are caused by the same imbalance in Yin and Yang, and a physician must be aware of and able to treat both. The theory and practice of acupuncture rarely distinguishes between physical and psychological diseases. Acupuncturists treat the entire person, often finding the causes of emotional upset in subtle physiological disturbances. Second, the tradition that the acupuncturist inherits is one of self-sacrifice, not only toward emperors, but toward any patient who seeks help. China's half-million acupuncturists are living examples of the Confucian belief in righteousness before profit, although not to the extent that cost Wen Chi his life.

Death by beheading or boiling in oil was not the worst punishment meted out in old China. Torture was a popular way of dealing with criminals and others from about 1100 to 200 B.C. Five types of punishment were fashionable during those centuries: branding on the forehead; cutting off the nose; cutting off ears, hands, feet, and kneecaps; castration; and execution by hanging, beheading, or boiling oil.

Breaking petty laws frequently resulted in a scar on the wrongdoer's forehead. Theft and harming someone else's travel coaches or clothes often led to having a nose cut off. Burglary and mutilation of city gates or bridges would cost the culprit an ear, or hand, or kneecap. Adultery and kidnapping, as well as robbery that ended in someone's death, were punishable by castration. So were certain kinds of treason. Death was reserved for those who committed murder or displeased the emperor in some way. And in what must seem to members of Alcoholics Anonymous a rather extreme way to keep people off the bottle and on the wagon, drunkenness carried with it the death penalty.

Castration was not used exclusively as a punishment for crime. Eunuchs were provided for the empresses of China and their ladies in waiting by castrating servants, a practice common to many Oriental and Middle Eastern countries. The only operation attributed to Hua T'o that survived his death and the burning of his writings was his castration procedure, which remained popular until this century. Hua T'o was, in fact, the last surgeon known in China until the late seventh century. Rather than surgery, China turned to acupuncture and other healing arts, both because Hua T'o's work was destroyed and because the religions that infiltrated the nation along the silk routes and the Burma roads preached the sanctity of the human body. Considering the advanced stage of Hua T'o's techniques, it is likely that China would have become the foremost country in surgery as well as acupuncture and herbal medicine if his work had been carried on by the physicians who came after him.

The Han dynasty that fostered, then ended Hua T'o's brilliant work in surgery also gave birth to another great physician, whose medical writings did survive. Through them he became known in China, in other Far Eastern countries, and in Europe, as "the Hippocrates of the East."

Chang Chung-ching was the first Chinese physician to compile and arrange the known works of medicine and set down a wide range of diagnostic techniques and treatments for common ailments. Chang was born in what is now the administrative district of Nanyang in Honan province sometime between 158 and 166 A.D. He studied medicine under Chang Pai-tsu, another native of Honan. Dr. Chang became so eminent that the Emperor Ling Ti bestowed upon him the Hiao Lien, or Master Graduate degree. Ling Ti, who ruled between 168 and 188 A.D., also made Chang administrative officer of the Changsha district of Hunan province, a powerful position in Han China.

Chang Chung-ching's major work was the *Shang-han Lun*, or *Treatise on Fevers*. It dealt with ailments the doctor believed were caused by exposure to cold. In another form, called *Shang-han Tsa-ping Lun,* Chang's treatise is still used by Chinese doctors as a basic text in general medicine. Centuries after Chang's death, doctors divided the *Shang-han Lun* into two parts, the first dealing with diagnosis and called by the name Dr. Chang gave it, and the second listing prescriptions, most of them composed of herbs, called the *Chin-Kuel Yao-lio Fang,* or *Prescriptions of the Golden Chamber.* In these and all his works, Chang stressed the theory that the human body is a composite of Yin and Yang forces. He divided symptoms and diseases into the two categories, exactly as the Chinese theory of the universe dictated. More than any doctor in the Han period, Chang was responsible through his support of Yin-Yang theory for the survival and popularity of acupuncture.

Along with his groundwork in diseases caused by cold, Dr. Chang delved into dozens of other illnesses and wrote treatises on many of them. He did extensive studies on diabetes and medical problems peculiar to women, and among his prescriptions were drug compounds that retain their effectiveness to this day.

Medical men of other countries often used Chang's work as the basis for their own. The *Treatise on Fevers* was translated into Japanese in about 1700. In Japan it is known as the *Sho Kan-ron* and remains in considerable repute as a medical authority. In Vietnam, the greatest doctor of that region's history, Lan Ong, used ancient Chinese texts of the *Shang-han Lun, Nei Ching,* and *Pen Ts'ao* as the sources for his encyclopedia of medicine, the most complete medical dictionary ever written in Vietnamese. Chinese medical researchers in recent centuries have isolated many important medicines from the remedies that Chang Chung-ching prescribed, including ephedrine, the most widely used drug in the world for relief of asthma. Dr. Chang's remedy for asthma included it over seventeen hundred years ago.

The Han dynasty produced other skilled physicians, including Shun Yu-yi, who like Dr. Chang divided his time between medicine and civil service. Unlike Chang, Shun flirted with death at the hands of one of the Han emperors.

Shun Yu-yi's highest medical ability was in the field of diagnosis. The Imperial Court recognized his talent and granted him a great civil honor. Emperor Wen Ti named Shun the keeper of the granaries of Ts'i, with the title Tsang Chung, or Father Tsang. But the doctor did not enjoy imperial favor for long, because of a preference he had for certain patients. He would turn away people he disliked no matter how ill they seemed, and because of this he soon angered Emperor Wen Ti. The ruler reacted with typical royal rage to Shun's obstinacy: he ordered the doctor's limbs cut off.

Shun Yu-yi was not blessed with any sons to carry on the family name and tradition in medicine. He had five daughters, one of whom accompanied him to Wen Ti's court when the sentence of death was handed down. She pleaded with the emperor for her father's limbs, asking him to take her as a slave girl instead. Unused to this kind of devotion and courage on the part of a daughter, Wen Ti suspended the sentence and even abolished punishment by maiming for the rest of his reign. Shun Yu-yi left the court with his daughter and returned to the practice of medicine, stripped of his civil post. But his narrow escape from the gallows proved to be an ill omen.

Ten years later, after Dr. Shun became even more famous for his diagnostic skill, the warrior general Liou Tsiang-lu was defeated and his army scattered. Shun Yu-yi had worked for General Liou as his army's physician. He disappeared after Liou met death on the battlefield. Except for a lengthy, and important, report on his life's work, Dr. Shun was never heard from again.

The physician may have been captured and forced to write the report in exchange for his life, for it is different than any other medical text of the Han dynasty. Shun wrote it as a memoir, detailing the patients he treated, the diagnoses he made of their complaints, the drugs he prescribed, and the books he used as references. The illnesses he cured included cirrhosis of the liver, hernia, lumbago, peritonitis, lung congestion, abscesses, paralysis, and other recognizable ailments. Of the books his report mentioned, only the *Nei Ching* survives, and probably not in the form in which he used it.

One of the reasons Dr. Shun fell into disrepute may have been his medical outlook, which was unusual for the era. Shun developed a logical method of classifying, analyzing, and treating illness not unlike the one used in the West today. He followed the classical texts only when the facts in a specific case did not contradict the text's suggestions for treatment. During the Han dynasty the classics in all fields were becoming extremely popular. Their formalized thinking dominated China, especially the Imperial Court. Little room was left for imaginative medical men such as Shun Yu-yi.

Hua T'o, Chang Chung-ching and Shun Yu-yi were the most illustrious doctors of the Han dynasty, but two other, less famous men left a large imprint on Chinese medicine as it is practiced today.

Huang Fu-mi, who lived from 215 to 282 A.D., wrote a book called *Chia I Ching,* a study of acupuncture and moxabustion. While the new diagnostic and treatment methods of Shun Yu-yi were disregarded, acupuncture continued to gain favor with the people. Wang Shu-ho, born at the very end of the Han era, authored the *Mo-ching*, a treatise on pulse diagnosis. Chinese acupuncturists and herb specialists study the pulse to discover the cause of illness. They consider it the foremost method of unearthing the true seat of disease, whatever a patient's symptoms may be. The *Mo-ching* was translated into Japanese, Tibetan, Arabic, and Persian, and found its way to the Middle East and Europe. Two works on pulse diagnosis were published in German in the seventeenth century, one in Frankfurt (1682)and the other in Nuremberg (1686). Both relied heavily on the *Mo-ching.* In 1735 Wang Shu-ho's theories, which were expansions on concepts set down in the *Nei Ching*, reached France in the writings of Pere du Halde under the title *Secret du pouls.* An earlier anonymous work, probably written by a Jesuit missionary in Canton, was published in Grenoble, France, in 1706. It was called the *Secrets de la médicine des chinois*, and created enough of a stir to be translated almost immediately into Italian and English. Much of it dwelled on the amazing ability of Chinese doctors to diagnose illness by feeling their patients' pulses.

After the classic forms of medicine were codified and expanded in the Han dynasty, the swell of Taoism throughout China insured that they would become the basis of modern acupuncture and herb medicine. Taoism taught the concepts of Yin and Yang, as interpreted by Lao Tzu, as the proper basis for conducting life. The people did not have to forego their strong belief in ancestor worship to accept the Taoist creed, or forsake the ancient classics they held dear. The Taoists found that they could modify these beliefs and still command the attention of China's masses without offending the traditions that the people regarded as vital to their lives.

Taoism reached its zenith between the third and seventh centuries. In many ways, so did traditional Chinese medicine, for during that period great doctors found remarkably effective cures for serious illnesses and excellent scholars rewrote and improved the classics of medicine. Emperors realized the worth of the prominent physicians and supported medical research and teaching.

The most famous doctor of the Taoist era was one of its earliest, Ko Hung. Ko was born in Kiangsu province, and came to medicine only after working as a carpenter to earn enough money for writing materials. He studied under Ko Huan, his uncle, who spent his own life searching for an elixir that would insure immortality. Ko Hung became a noted scholar, and along the way earned a reputation as a capable military leader. In 302 A.D. he led the emperor's forces that squashed the rebellion of Shih Ping. As a reward he was named military advisor to the Governor of Canton, but soon resigned to take up an ascetic's life in the Lo Fu Mountains. There he could follow his uncle's lead in searching for a key to eternal life.

Ko became an alchemist, as did many Taoist doctors, and under the name Pao P'u-tzu wrote a book on alchemy, magic, and dietetics, one of the finest works of the Taoist period. But his major contribution to Chinese life rests on two medical treatises, one a book of medications, the other a list of first-aid treatments.

Ko Hung believed that man could do much to prevent disease by taking good care of himself physically. An entire chapter of his first book discusses methods of keeping fit while going about the daily business of living. Ko advocated good eating habits, similar to the ones doctors prescribe today, and careful attention to getting enough, but not too much, sleep. He developed a breathing technique that allowed the proper flow of Ch'i through the body. And he brilliantly described and categorized dozens of diseases.

Ko was the first doctor in the world to write about smallpox, five centuries before an account in Arabic was set down. He accurately portrayed beriberi, hepatitis, bubonic plague, acute lymphangitis, and rabies. He also discovered the early signs of leprosy and distinguished them from similar warnings that indicate other diseases.

For all his scientific work, Ko Hung never lost his fascination for potions that would yield eternal life. He worked out a formula for immortality that contained gold, mercury, jade, sulphur, cinnabar, and yellow arsenic. While it is likely that he took the elixir himself, it did little good in keeping him alive beyond a normal life span. He died at the age of eighty-one but, according to legend, his body was very light when the pallbearers picked it up, as though only the shell remained and the rest had escaped death to live on into eternity.

Another Taoist doctor, Sun Szu-miao, did not choose to seek eternal life. Born in Shensi province in 581 A.D., Sun began studying the Taoist classics written by Lao Tzu and Chuang Tzu at age seven. He became a respected and sought-after scholar, and was summoned twice from his retreat in the Tapo Mountains to the Imperial Court. Each time he refused offers of high positions, claiming illness, and returned to his meditations.

Sun used his time in the mountains to write thirty volumes on medical theory and practice. Two brought him immediate fame: *Chien Chin Yao Fang,* or *The Thousand Golden Prescriptions;* and *Chien Chin I Fang*, or *Another Thousand Golden Prescriptions.* He also wrote treatises on emotional happiness, hygiene, ophthalmology, and sex (this last called *In the Depth of the Pillow*).

Between writing books, Sun developed striking techniques for treating illness. The most famous, which establishes the Chinese as the first people to use inoculations and serum therapy, was Sun's procedure for treating smallpox victims. He took dried fluid from a patient's sores and injected it under the skin of active pustules. The remedy worked and became popular throughout China and, much later, in the Middle East and Europe.

The doctor showed his brilliant insight when he attributed tuberculosis to a tiny creature that ate away the lung of its victim. Sun also categorized tumors into five different types, and developed treatments for all of them.

Dr. Sun's eminence grew until he was given the name *chen jen*, or man of wisdom, by Emporor Tai Tsung in 660 A.D. His methods became so popular among the people that since his death they have called him Yao Wang, King of Medicine. The Communist government recently issued a postage stamp commemorating Sun's contributions to the masses, and in 1962 the Academy of Medicine in Peking held a ceremonial tribute to him. Until the Communist revolution in 1949, his birthday was celebrated as a national holiday. Sun Szu-miao lived to the ripe old age of 101 without the benefit of Ko Hung's immortality potion, which kept the latter alive only to the age of eighty-one.

Another prominent doctor whose face adorns a postage stamp was Shen Kua, a man of many and diverse talents. Shen was an expert in architecture, agriculture, history, medicine, and astronomy. In about 1070 A.D. he proclaimed that the sun revolved around the earth not in a circle, as had been thought, but in an ellipse. In the West, Johannes Kepler, the great German astronomer, reached nearly the same conclusion at the beginning of the seventeenth century.

These practitioners of the healing arts give only an inkling of the richness of Chinese medical history. Today's acupuncturist, whether trained before the Communist revolution in the classic way, or after it in modern medical schools, has a long and illustrious heritage to uphold. Every Son of Han, as the Chinese have been called, knows this; the Chinese people venerate no fewer than eighty-seven doctors as great men. Combined with the emphasis on ethical behavior that permeates Chinese life, the acupuncturist is a man to be respected and trusted.

Another thread in the history of Chinese medicine helps the acupuncturist keep the high regard he has held since he first began using needles made out of stone. Nearly all the great Chinese physicians of antiquity built their medical prowess on the works of doctors who preceded them. The influence of history on modern medicine aligns with the Chinese belief in the durability and worth of ancient customs. The people do not believe that the acupuncturist is a magician who uses strange materials in odd ways. His techniques come from the ancients, just as Chinese life comes from the ancient philosophers' ways of living. The people view their history the same way the acupuncturist views his. A line of communication, grounded in forty centuries of experience, opens between the masses of people and the physicians. It is a line that began before the written memory of man, with China's legendary emperors.

Two ancient gods of the Chinese people began the arts of acupuncture and herbal therapy. The lives of Huang Ti and Shen Nung are couched in legend. That they existed has not been proven, but neither has it been proven that they did not. To the Chinese people, and to the acupuncturist in his village shop, their reality goes beyond written evidence or artifacts dug from the ground. It hangs on the undeniable truth of lives saved and misery alleviated. Shen Nung and Huang Ti were the second and third of the Three August Emperors, preceded by Fu Hsi, the legendary discoverer of the Pa Kua.

Shen Nung created herbal therapy, or so it is said. He was endowed with an unusual characteristic that enabled him to test the effects of herbs on himself: a transparent stomach. So great was his ability to discover herb remedies that he took as many as seventy poisons in one day and then found the antidotes for them. Emperor Shen is revered as the founder of agriculture and dentistry as well as herb medicine.

In the course of his experiments on himself, Shen Nung (whose name means Divine Agriculturist) compounded 365 remedies for illness, forty from minerals, sixty-eight from animals, and the rest from plants. They were of three types: nontoxic, semitoxic, and poisonous. The nontoxic drugs were considered superior to the others, and the poisonous drugs were used only when all else failed.

Shen Nung reigned from 3737 to 2697 B.C., before the time even the most enthusiastic Chinese historians place the invention of writing. No edition of the *Pen Ts'ao*, the pharmacopoeia containing Shen Nung's prescriptions, survives from that time, and it is doubtful that any was written then. But the number of drugs in the book provides a clue to when the work was actually set down.

During the Han dynasty, the ancient Chinese number systems became popular in all walks of life. The 365 remedies of the *Pen Ts'ao* corresponded to the days of the year in number, a likely type of correlation for the Han era. A writer of the time, who preferred to remain unknown and to use Shen Nung's name, compiled the *Pen Ts'ao* that has served as a basis for herbal medicine. Another doctor, who lived in the Taoist period, T'ao Hung-ching, supposedly had the original text written by Shen Nung and published an annotated edition of it called the *Ming I Pie Lu*. Dr. T'ao wrote his commentaries in black ink to contrast with the red ink used by Shen Nung. Shen Nung was called the Blazing Emperor because he ruled China with fire, and the color red was often associated with him.

For twelve centuries the *Ming I Pie Lu* was unknown except in legend. At the end of the Ming dynasty (about 1600 A.D.), the introduction to T'ao's work was found in a cave at Tun huang, China, along with other relics of the Taoist times. Archaeological excavations now being carried out in China may yet shed new light on this, and other, legends.

T'ao Hung-ching was himself a man of many accomplishments and has been called the Leonardo da Vinci of China. Born in 452 A.D. near Tanyang, on the banks of the Yellow River, T'ao became an astronomer, mathematician, calligrapher, alchemist, and doctor. After serving as tutor to the sons of Emperor Kao Ti of the Ch'i dynasty, T'ao followed the tradition of other scholars and retired to the mountains to study and write. He built a three-story straw hut and installed China's first planetarium on the top floor.

The unknown writer of Han and T'ao Hung-ching were but the first two of many writers to revise the *Pen Ts'ao*. At least twenty-four later versions of the work are known, including the one still used by Chinese doctors. Called the *Pen Ts'ao Chang Mu*, it was written in 1593 by Dr. Li Shih-chen.

Li Shih-chen's pharmacopeoia contains 1,892 drugs and 10,000 prescriptions. Li classified the drugs into sixteen divisions and sixty-two classes according to their biological characteristics and value as remedies. He spent twenty-seven years compiling the book, which included the opinions and conclusions of at least five hundred different authors. While he may not have approved of all the remedies he listed, he left the choice up to future readers. The *Pen Ts'ao Chang Mu* recommends a dried and grated heart from a white horse as a cure for forgetfulness and the ashes of a skull (presumably an animal's) mixed with water and taken before bedtime as a soothing potion to relieve restlessness and hysteria. But along with the more arcane remedies are thousands that have proven effective in treating many serious diseases, most of them mixtures of common Chinese herbs (see Chapter X).

The *Pen Ts'ao Chang Mu* did not discuss only medical matters. Chapters dealt with geography, history, philosophy, chemistry, foods, and the art of good living. One part of the encyclopedia set down four simple rules for maintaining happiness and health. Called "The Art of Acquiring a Long and Healthy Life," it suggested that people:

1. Control the emotions of the heart;
2. Moderate the intake of food and drink;
3. Perform daily work according to a plan and system;
4. Follow definite rules for rest and sleep.

Li's *Pen Ts'ao* mentions many diseases that had become common in China, including syphilis, which was brought to the East in 1504 A.D. by colonists who settled in Canton. The medical encyclopedia was translated into every Oriental language and found its way to many European countries. Its contents formed the basis for a number of Western medical techniques.

In dentistry, Li Shih-chen gave the formula for the silver paste still used to fill cavities. He divided the paste into its ingredients—silver, mercury, and tin—and told the exact proportion needed to make the mixture harden properly. Although the first written formula for the paste is in the *Pen Ts'ao,* its use in China was common as early as the fifth century A.D. It did not become popular in Europe until after 1815.

Shen Nung's legacy, legendary or real, became the skeleton for a vast body of medical literature. It influenced generation after generation of doctors, including those of today. Shen Nung is revered throughout the Orient, with temples in his honor still standing in places like Hanoi, North Vietnam. There North Vietnamese doctors held three feasts a year as late as 1954. The main altar in the temple has three memorials, to Fu Hsi, Shen Nung, and Huang Ti. As the father of acupuncture, it is fitting that Huang Ti, the Yellow Emperor, stands next to Fu Hsi and Shen Nung.

Huang Ti, legend has it, took the helm of China from Shen Nung in 2697 B.C. He was a man of great wisdom, endowed with the ability to study nature and transfer what he discerned to the practical world of men. Once while he was gazing at the stars his attention became fixed on the Big Dipper constellation. From its shape he envisioned a two-wheeled vehicle that would carry men or heavy burdens. He ordered the construction of China's first rickshaw and built a park where people could go to ride in the carts. He created a system of musical notes and designed instruments on which to play them. He instituted ritual into Chinese life and ruled by sophisticated civil laws. And he authored, or formulated, the classic of Chinese medicine that is responsible for nearly all Chinese medical theory and practice.

In discussion with his chief minister and doctor, Ch'i Po, Huang Ti thrashed out the complexities of the human body, always demonstrating how the Chinese theory of the universe works inside man. The conclusions and principles of anatomy, medicine, and health that Huang Ti and Ch'i Po formulated were written down in the *Nei Ching,* more formally called the *Huang Ti Nei Ching Su Wen*, the *Yellow Emperor's Classic of Internal Medicine.*

As with Shen Nung and the *Pen Ts'ao,* it is impossible to establish Huang Ti as the actual author of the *Nei Ching.* Many tales are told about Huang Ti's life, most of them not within the realm of believability. His mother, Fu Pao, supposedly gave birth to him on the bank of a river after he was miraculously conceived. At the end of his one-hundred-year reign, the phoenix, a bird beloved by the Chinese people, appeared for the first time. So did the Ch'i lin, a strange animal somewhat like the unicorn in appearance. Both attested to the greatness of Huang Ti.

The *Nei Ching* is divided into two parts. The first, *Su Wen,* or *Simple Questions,* contains the principles of medicine and interprets the theory of the universe as it pertains to health. The second, *Ling Shu,* or *Magic Gate,* tells the actual ways an acupuncturist may prevent and cure illness. The theories of the first part and the practices of the second part still form the foundation of Chinese medicine.

The *Nei Ching* was far ahead of its time in medical theory, even by Western standards. It revealed that the blood circulates in a continous system of vessels, and likened it to a nerve-ending circle. The West reached the same conclusion as long as two thousand years after the Chinese discovery. For the most part, the *Nei Ching* prescribes only cures aimed at restoring harmony within the human being. But in drastic cases, such as malignant tumors, the book recommends surgery. The functions of the organs are explored in intricate detail, and illnesses accompanied by fevers are scrutinized extensively.

The text of Huang Ti's classic can be traced only to the Early Han dynasty, and then only in references made by physicians in their own works. In the basic form known today, it was compiled by Wang Ping of the Tang dynasty. His 762 A.D. edition of the work claimed that he had access to Huang Ti's original manuscript, but no proof has been found that he did. It is more likely that Wang Ping used commentaries made by many physicians to form his edition. The *Nei Ching* has always enjoyed the favor of China's emperors, and in the Sung dynasty Wang Ping's edition was revised under imperial order. It survives from that time, about 1200A.D., with few changes.

At least forty-nine editions of the *Nei Ching* were written before the Sung version. It is still pertinent and usable as a medical text because it underwent constant revision based on centuries of experience. It has retained its original form of a dialogue between emperor and minister because of the Chinese distaste for abstractions and respect for the ability of ancient men.

This respect is instilled in the modern acupuncturist as he studies the contents of the classical works. In the *Pen Ts'ao* and *Nei Ching*, the village physician finds both treatments and reasons for illness. The people he sees venerate the ancient men who may have originated those techniques and principles. The search for health is common to all manner of Chinese people—emperors or peasants—and has gone on since the beginnings of civilization.

Respect for the ancient emperors and ways is not the only reason the people of China prefer to be treated by acupuncture. They have a better one: acupuncture works. And herbal medicine has been providing excellent cures for too many centuries to be ignored. The people feel it works because acupuncture shares a common stem with the other petals of the Chinese cultural flower. That stem, the Chinese theory of the universe, has been most useful to the people. Through forty centuries of cruel emperors, bloody wars, and savage invasions, it has kept the Chinese race alive.

CHAPTER IV

YIN AND YANG: APPLIED THEORY IN ACUPUNCTURE

As heaven is round and the earth square, so a man's head is round and the foot square. As heaven has its sun and moon, its order of stars, rain and wind, thunder and lightning, so man has two eyes, a set of teeth, joy and anger, voice and sound. The earth with its mountains and valleys, rocks and stones, trees and shrubs, weeds and grasses, has its parallel on the human body in the shoulders and armpits, nodes and tuberosities, tendons and muscles, hairs and down. The four limbs correspond with the four seasons, the twelve joints with the twelve months. The pulse is of twelve different kinds to agree with the twelve rivers. The human skeleton has 360 bones for the simple reason that there are the same number of degrees in a circle.

—Chinese Medical History

WHEN CHIANG Kai-shek and the Kuomintang were in power in China, Western medicine was fostered and grew in popularity with the common people. Missionary doctors operated in China's interior with Generalissimo Chiang's blessings, bringing the "new" methods of healing the sick to millions who had experienced only

57

acupuncture and herb medicine. Chinese doctors, eager to please the whims of the people, began to study Western medical theory and techniques. Chiang's opposition, the Communist forces led by Mao Tse-tung, were in closer contact with the masses and sensed that traditional medicine was the real wish of most of the people. The Communists supported the "old" medicine.

Many Chinese doctors who took up the study of Western medicine had no real desire to forsake the ancient healing arts. They did it to avoid being labeled Communist and risking a stay in the notorious Kuomintang detention camps. It was easier to comply with the Generalissimo's wishes, bolstered as they were by the pressure of the United States government and John D. Rockefeller's endowment of the Peking University Medical Center.

Western medicine demanded a knowledge of anatomy in Western terms. This, in turn, required dissection of human bodies to see how they functioned, a standard part of any Western doctor's training. But dissection posed a real problem, for the Chinese people believe that the body must remain intact, even after death, for the person to take his proper place among the revered ancestors. Few families were willing to donate the corpse of a loved one for medical students to practice on, and the cause of Western medicine faltered.

Chiang Kai-shek came up with a solution. Kuomintang authorities would ship the bodies of newly-deceased concentration camp prisoners to hospitals and the P.U.M.C. for use in anatomy classes. Arrangements were made, and within weeks a shipment of cadavers arrived in Peking. But when the anatomy instructors saw them, they were disappointed. The corpses were mutilated; the prisoners had been executed by beheading. Hospital officials told the Kuomintang that they were grateful for their help, but bodies without heads could not be used to teach anatomy. The Kuomintang responded with a simple change in procedure. They ordered the camp commanders to strangle their prisoners to death rather than behead them. Anatomy classes soon resumed.

Generalissimo Chiang and the Kuomintang fell from power for this and many other reasons. But even during the war-torn years before Mao's People's Army drove Chiang into exile on Formosa, a majority of the Chinese people stayed with their *chung i,* traditional physicians, rather than go to *hsi i,* the Western-style doctors.

Although the traditional physicians of China have never had the benefit of dissection classes, they have always had a clear idea of the human anatomy, handed down through many generations. Their knowledge is sufficient to allow the successful practice of medicine, even though their analysis of the human body has been proven wrong in certain instances. The discrepancies do not matter. Chinese medicine developed independently of Western medicine, has a different philosophy as its foundation, and a theory of how the body works that largely contradicts Western ideas. As long as it proves to be an effective basis for curing illness, which it has for thousands of years, the Chinese concept of anatomy serves its primary, and highest, purpose.

To the Westerner listening in on Huang Ti's discourse with Chi Po, their words will sound like nothing more than the mystical utterings of witches exchanging spells. Illness is explained in terms of disharmony between man and nature, and, in man, between Yin and Yang. When the two ancients discuss a disease that is probably malaria, Huang Ti says:

> The chill and fever are due to the alternating replacement of the Yang and Yin. The phenomenon is brought about by the contraction of heat in summer. This heat is stored up beneath the skin

and will manifest itself in the form of chills and fever at other seasons when the Yang and Yin lose their state of counterbalance.

This is hardly what the West would call a "scientific" explanation for malaria. Yet for a Chinese physician schooled in the classic manner, it is enough to show him the way to successful treatment of the malaria-ridden patient. The acupuncturist will combine these words of Huang Ti with the principles of Chinese anatomy and physiology as the *Nei Ching* first set them down. He will choose the points on the body that produce the desired effect when his needles are twisted into them. The *Nei Ching* also tells him how to do this, in specific terms that cover every known malady. But before the Chinese physician can translate the principles of treatment into action, he must understand how, according to the *Nei Ching,* the human body works.

Yin and Yang, the dual expressions of Ch'i, are as important in medicine as in the Chinese theory of the universe. Ch'i is what the Chinese call the motivating force behind all life. All matter is made of Yin and Yang, including every part of the human body. Illnesses are either Yin or Yang and the therapy used to cure them will be either Yin or Yang. The parts of the body that are Yin follow the concept of Yin as yielding, negative, and feminine. Those that are Yang are dominating, positive, and masculine. Diseases follow the same pattern. So do treatments, although to treat a Yin disease, the acupuncturist will often use a Yang technique. The reason goes back to the flow of Ch'i through the body.

The undefinable and invisible force of life that the Chinese believe exists is the true basis of traditional medicine. Ch'i comes into the body at birth and leaves at death. During a person's lifetime it flows in a specific and continuous pattern in the forms of Yin and Yang.

Ch'i does not inhabit the body at random, although it is present throughout the organism. Instead it flows inside a system of channels called "meridians" that extend into the arms and legs and around the torso beneath the surface of the skin. These meridians are not the vessels of the circulatory system that carry blood. They are not the nerves familiar to Western medicine. Until a few years ago, they were thought to exist only in the minds of Chinese physicians, and Western doctors scoffed at the idea. But research in Korea, France, and the U.S.S.R. has proven that the channels do indeed exist.

Acupuncturists have always believed that the meridians existed. Chinese doctors in the 1920's and 1930's witnessed postmortem dissections in Peking and were presented with the visible lack of the meridians. They ignored the evidence, very wisely. Not only does their form of medicine work, but to question that the Ch'i meridians are there means also to deny the truth of the Chinese theory of the universe. That a doctor of traditional medicine—and most other Chinese people—will never do. It would mean surrendering the beliefs upon which Chinese civilization was founded and has thrived, and an immense loss of face.

Even Mao Tse-tung, whose supreme power in China has been indisputable for the last quarter-century, decided not to affront the people's choice of traditional medicine. He had extremely practical reasons. After the successful communist takeover in 1949, Mao had to keep his promise of taking care of the people or lose the faith of China's masses. He himself had turned to Western medicine and stayed with it until his illness in 1952 forced him to seek a cure from traditional doctors. Even if that did not restore his faith in acupuncture and herb medicine, the medical care situation in China did. There were at the time 420,000 traditional doctors and fewer than thirty thousand Western physicians. Only traditional medical care could be provided for the millions of peasants the revolution had liberated. Practicality overshadowed whatever Mao's opinion of Yin-Yang theory, Ch'i, and the needles of acupuncture might have been. As proof of the effectiveness of acupuncture mounted in the '50's and '60's, the Chairman's earlier proclamation of it as the true "medicine of the people" earned him even greater stature among the masses. Just as the acupuncturist ignores the physical invisibility of the meridians, Mao Tse-tung ignored the contradiction of using a medical system based on a philosophy that holds the individual in high esteem and at the same time ruling by socialist principles. Even the politically indoctrinated acupuncturists trained in modern medical schools must learn the classic theories in order to practice traditional medicine. Although he has slashed China's cultural heritage at its roots in many ways, Mao may be keeping it alive at the same time. Every acupuncture needle that finds its way into a meridian of Ch'i carries with it the message of China's ancient theory of the universe. The seed of Chinese culture may yet endure beyond Mao's, or any, communist government.

Mao Tse-tung's method of keeping his influence strong among the people exactly parallels one of the basic precepts of traditional medicine. Modern Chinese workers are urged to find solutions to difficult problems by reading Mao's words and following the path of his wisdom. Traditional medical theory tells the people to seek harmony by achieving Tao, the Supreme Way. It would appear that Chairman Mao's power rests less on the theories of Karl Marx than on transferring the force of life from the Ch'i of the Chinese theory of the universe to his own words. History alone will reveal if his words can supplant the four-thousand-year-old belief in Tao and Ch'i. It is certain, however, that the Chinese way of thinking, which makes acupuncture possible, is far from obsolete.

Part of that way of thinking is that man is a replica of the universe, and that the flow of Ch'i through his body corresponds to the movement of the force of life in larger segments of nature. The seasons, climate, and time of day influence the flow and play a vital role in maintaining and restoring health. The seasons and months of the year are either Yin or Yang, and Yin or Yang illnesses are likely to occur when their part of the duality is at its zenith.

Ch'i is not presently in the body in the same quantity at all times, or evenly distributed throughout the human organs. As Yin and Yang it fluctuates, pulsing through the human being the way the seasons pulsate in the rhythm of nature. The first principle of medicine a Chinese physician must learn is the relationship between Yin and Yang in the body. Yin and Yang may not be equal—one rises as the other falls—but their total amount must be properly distributed among the organs for the body to remain healthy. In any organ, Yin and Yang are delicately balanced with each other. Illness results if the balance is disrupted. At certain times of the day, the Yin or Yang "influence" will be stronger than its counterpart, but this is a normal rhythm and will not cause illness or disease. When an imbalance causes sickness, the acupuncturist tries to discover where Yin or Yang has become too strong and with his needles restore the balance, as prescribed in the *Nei Ching*. The illness disappears when he has done this successfully.

The Chinese theory of the universe taught that Yin and Yang produced the Five Elements, and from them all matter was fashioned. The Chinese mind—unflawed by logical processes—reasoned that the human body was no exception, and that the elements must have their parallels in the human anatomy. The elements were conceived of as functions rather than inert substances, a view of matter that Western science now accepts. The organs of the body, which the Chinese rightly saw as useless *except* in their functions, must directly correlate with the elements, since man is a microcosm of the universe. The Chinese medical system, always aimed at finding the internal root of illness, could progress another step.

Wood, fire, earth, metal, and water correspond to the liver, heart, spleen, lungs, and kidneys respectively, according to Chinese medical theory. They are the *Ts'ang,* or solid organs. They dwell inside the body where Yin, the dark, internal principle predominates, and their functions are internal. Therefore they are subject to all the Yin characteristics.

Each of the solid organs has a corresponding hollow organ. These are called *Fu.* They are, in order, the gallbladder, small intestine, stomach, large intestine, and bladder. Unlike the *Ts'ang* organs, which, like winter, store substances, the *Fu* organs, or viscera, eliminate substances, much as summer does. They are Yang in functions and characteristics.

The *Ts'ang* organs and *Fu* viscera govern how the body will work. The liver, heart, spleen, lungs, and kidneys are the instigators of all movement in the body, and the *Fu* viscera are directed by them. Each of the *Ts'ang* organs has specific attributes of its own, often corresponding to interactions between the seasons, natural forces, or men rather than medical function. The Chinese based their system of anatomy and physiology on what they saw in the world, often making it sound more like mysticism than medicine.

Lacking the inclination to prove their theories by logical reasoning, early Chinese doctors used the weight of parallelisms as conclusive evidence. They drew on the correspondencies, extended to medical matters, and on the ways people function in social situations and government. The parallels could be drawn because the Tao that ruled nature and man also dictated how government and business should be conducted. The correspondencies made the system fit into the theory of the universe and, with the law of Yin and Yang, enabled the physician to intuitively discern the functions of the organs and viscera.

Once he knew the characteristics and function of each organ, the acupuncturist could find the proper way to treat it when an imbalance in Yin and Yang caused a malfunction. Relying on the Chinese number system, he began assigning characteristics by finding the number one organ that corresponded with the number one element, wood.

The physician decided that the first organ is the liver, which is the seat of anger and stores the blood. It has a rancid odor, sour taste, and brown color in the correspondencies. The liver opens to the outside by way of the eyes and produces tears. It feeds the nails and, with the flowing system of the "fives," generates the heart, just as wood creates fire. It regulates the lungs, which would destroy it if allowed to run independently, in the same way as metal (the element of the lungs) destroys wood.

In society, the liver is represented by a general whose duty it is to direct operations on a battlefield. The body's vital fluids are filtered through the liver. Those that are needed go on to the lungs; those that are no longer useful are eliminated through the gallbladder, the liver's corresponding viscerus.

The liver became the first organ because, like its element wood, it is unusual in characteristics and function. Wood is a living element, the outer covering of growing plants. The other elements make up the inanimate objects in the universe, but wood is reserved for living things. The harmonious flow of the elements begins with wood, so that all substances can be traced to it. The liver's function in the body is equally important, a fact well known to Western as well as Chinese doctors.

Modern scientific research disclosed that the body's metabolism is controlled by the liver, just as traditional Chinese medical theory states. All other organs are secondary in that respect. The lungs, for example, take in oxygen that eventually fuels the liver, and the heart, no more than a pump, circulates the enriched blood to the liver. But it is the liver that dictates the rate at which other organs perform their jobs and maintains the proper flow of nourishment to every part of the body. Billions of cells in the body undergo chemical changes that create energy. The energy is used to produce new material that replaces dead cells. The liver regulates this creative process and starts the chain reaction that eventually yields a living human being. Although they did not know the scientific reasons for its importance, the ancient Chinese, armed only with intuition and perception, realized that the liver was vital to the welfare of the sophisticated human organism. Once again their theory of the universe opened the gate to an amazing accurate conclusion about the nature of life.

Chinese medical philosophy perceived the other organs in much the same way. The heart, corresponding to the element fire, smells like toast, has a bitter taste, deep red color, and is the seat of happiness. It contains the spirit of man and stores the pulse. The heart produces blood, generates the spleen, and controls the kidneys. Its opening is the tongue and its fluid is perspiration. It feeds the skin. Its *Fu* correspondent is the small intestine.

The heart functions as an emperor does in society. Wisdom and insight emanate from within it. Along with the liver, the heart guides man's conduct toward woman. A Chinese man in love will often say to his sweetheart, "I give you my heart and my liver." According to Chinese anatomy, the heart has three chambers.

The organ of the earth is the spleen. It is yellow, tastes sweet, and has a fragrant odor. The spleen is the center of thought and stores the body's nutrition, just as the earth stores man's food. It corresponds to the stomach and along with it acts as the keeper of the royal granaries—sentries guarding the emperor's storehouses.

The spleen produces flesh and controls the liver. It creates and directs the five tastes and aids in digestion. Its external opening is the mouth and its fluid is saliva.

The spleen generates the lungs, which correspond to the element metal (sometimes translated as air). The lungs have a hot taste, white color, and smell like raw fish. They store energy and are the center of sorrow. Their *Fu* correspondent is the large intestine and they supply nourishment to the skin. On the outside of the body, they are visible as the nose and they produce the nasal secretions. The function of the lungs is compared to that of civil administrators: they keep order in the body.

The fifth and last of the *Ts'ang* organs are the kidneys. They are black, taste salty, and have a putrid odor. Human will lives inside them and they are the seat of all fears. They generate the liver and control the spleen. The kidneys act with great efficiency, like a secretary of labor who uses intelligence to control strength. They correspond to the element water and are related to the gallbladder.

According to Chinese medical theory, two more organs dwell inside the body. They are called the "Triple Warmer" and the "Gate of Life." Both have caused consternation among Chinese and Western doctors, but both are still used in the practice of acupuncture.

The Triple Warmer, or the "Three Burning Spaces," as the Chinese name for it is sometimes translated, defies accurate definition. The *Nei Ching* considers it a human sewage system, but gives it no definite form. Other sources ascribe to it the ability to motivate the vital fluids between the various solid and hollow organs, and still others claim that the Triple Warmer is the link between man and the universe.

Chinese physicians agree on one property of the Triple Warmer: it assists in the regulation of the other organs. The top third of it, or the upper burning space, keeps food from leaving the stomach. The middle burning space aids digestion in the small intestine and spurs the products of the digestive process to the lungs. It also watches over the large intestine, liver, spleen, and bladder. The lower burning space is responsible for the excretion of waste matter.

The Triple Warmer is a Yin organ. Related to society, it is like the official in charge of rivers, lakes, and streams. Even today, when modern science has adequately proven that the burning spaces do not exist, traditional physicians insist that they are there. They are vital to the acupuncturist, who cannot cure some illnesses without them. Many serious diseases are treated by changing the Yin-Yang balance in the Triple Warmer. The acupuncturist's proof of their existence is simply that he can cure those illnesses ascribed to the burning spaces. Doctors trained in both Chinese and Western medicine compare the Triple Warmer's function to that of the lymphatic system, which would allow for cures by acupuncture.

The Gate of Life provides even more confusion. It is Yang and rests between the kidneys. In the male it produces semen and in the female performs the function of the uterus. Chinese doctors see no difficulty in proclaiming that the male and female sex organs are the same except in function. The theory of Yin and Yang provides the reason: man is Yang and woman is Yin, and since the theory is basically sexual, the difference will obviously show up in the reproductive organs. The

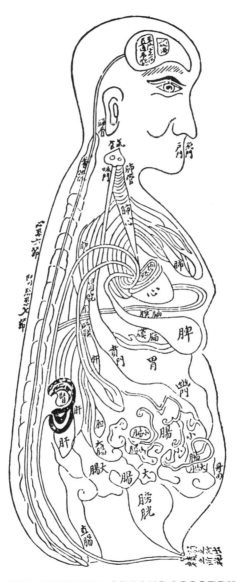

FIG. 1 THE INTERNAL ORGANS ACCORDING TO CHINESE ANATOMY

fact that the male sex organ is productive and the female sex organ receptive further proves Yin-Yang theory to be correct.

Modern Chinese doctors identify the Gate of Life as the organ of Circulation-Sex. Both it and the Triple Warmer are identified by function rather than structure. The Triple Warmer circulates nervous energy and warmth and the Gate of Life moves the blood and sexual fluids.

The Gate of Life may be compared to an ambassador of happiness and joy. It is as important to the practice of acupuncture as the Triple Warmer, and equally immune to any attempt at setting it right as an anatomical concept.

Early Chinese physicians made an even more flagrant error in their estimation of the brain. They considered it to be a small and rather insignificant organ, with little influence over the body. It was not a center of thought—the spleen was—and did not nearly fill the cranial cavity (see Figure 1).

These and other mistakes in the Chinese analysis of the human body (see Figures 2 through 13) stemmed from the unique Chinese philosophy of the universe. Doctors in ancient times reasoned that since the universe is in constant flux, the composition of the body means little compared to the way it works. They saw no reason to distinguish between anatomy and physiology, between structure and function. As with every part of their lives, the Chinese people cared less about *what* an organ was than *how* it helped produce a healthy, thriving individual. Only then could each organ's contribution to harmony be understood, and its balance of Yin and Yang restored if that harmony became upset.

The quirk of Chinese thinking that allows practicality without logic also makes possible effective medicine with a flawed knowledge of the human organism. Had dissection not been forbidden (there is some evidence that a few bodies were studied over the centuries, but it never became a regular or approved practice), the Chinese might have developed a medical system similar to the West's. Given their ability to observe and their amazing intuition, they may even have created a far superior one.

Instead, the Chinese performed an even harder task. They reduced the complex human body to factors that easily agreed with their philosophy, drew parallels between health, society, and nature, and invented a form of treatment, acupuncture, that did not depend on correct scientific knowledge. Acupuncture cures illness because it relies upon a single principle: man echoes nature. Nature is precise, therefore man is precise. The workings of nature can be systematically set down, and so can the physical workings of man. Predictable order reigns in nature and in man.

Man as a reflection of nature becomes vivid in the interaction of the *Ts'ang* organs or *Fu* viscera. Just as the elements create and destroy each other, the organs and viscera generate and limit each other. The order of

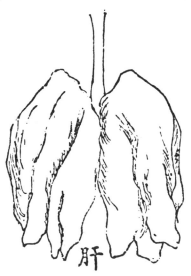

FIG. 2 THE LIVER

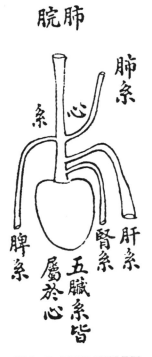

脘肺

肺系

系 心

脾系 腎系 肝系 五臟系皆 屬於心

FIG. 3 THE HEART

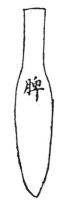

脾

FIG. 4 THE SPLEEN

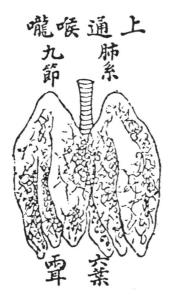

FIG. 5 THE LUNGS

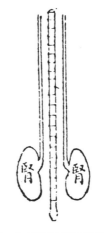

FIG. 6 THE KIDNEYS

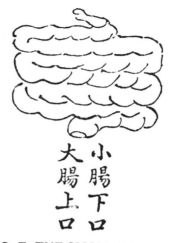

小腸下口
大腸上口

FIG. 7 THE SMALL INTESTINE

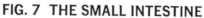

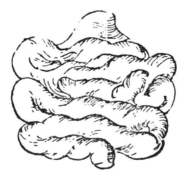

FIG. 8 THE LARGE INTESTINE

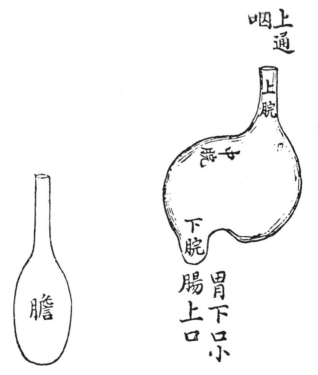

FIG. 9 THE GALLBLADDER   FIG. 10 THE STOMACH

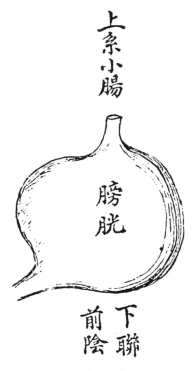

FIG. 11 THE BLADDER

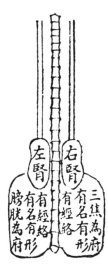

FIG. 12 THE TRIPLE WARMER (Three Burning Spaces)
       ORGAN

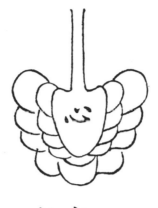

絡 包 心

FIG. 13 THE GATE OF LIFE, OR CIRCULATION-SEX ORGAN

their interaction is the same as that of the elements they correspond to, and the acupuncturist depends on the body to act as nature does. He sees seasonal disturbances as excesses of Yin or Yang, and illness in the same way. He uses his needles to move excess Yin or Yang from one place to another, restoring balance. He does not doubt the truth of the relationships of the organs any more than he would the relationships of the seasons. The universe is in harmony, therefore man must be. The system of medical correspondencies tells the acupuncturist exactly where harmony in the body has been disturbed and he directs his needles to that point. He knows the characteristics of the seasons, and the organs, intimately.

Since nature begins its rhythm in spring, the body begins its functions in the liver. The element wood parallels both. What begins in spring flourishes in summer, and the liver generates the heart, which corresponds to summer and fire. The heart generates the spleen, and summer flows into late summer (the extra season). Late summer and the spleen are represented by the element earth. Late summer becomes fall, so the spleen generates the lungs, and autumn and the lungs correspond to metal. Metal creates water, so the lungs generate the kidneys and winter overcomes fall.

The acupuncturist uses these relationships every time he treats a patient. Assume a patient contracts an illness in winter. The Chinese doctor searches for the seat of the illness in the body. He knows that in nature, a winter disturbance will be caused by something going awry in fall. Winter is the season of the kidneys, which is generated by the lungs, autumn's organ. The acupuncturist will seek the center of the illness in the patient's lungs, regardless of his symptoms. The lungs should show an imbalance of Yin and Yang. With his needles, the traditional physician will correct the imbalance, the flow of Ch'i will resume unhampered, and the illness will cease.

Although this example is highly oversimplified—many other factors must be considered before using the needles—it serves to demonstrate how the acupuncturist views the body in relation to nature and the seasons. He also knows that climatic conditions correspond to the seasons, elements, and organs. He takes into consideration heat, cold, wind, humidity, and dryness.

Excessive heat harms the heart; excessive cold injures the lungs. Too much wind will bring a disease to the liver, and too much humidity will cause an illness of the spleen. Extremely dry weather damages the kidneys. The climates interact as the seasons, elements, and organs do, and provide another clue to the location of a Yin-Yang imbalance.

After the acupuncturist considers the seasons, elements, climates, and organs, he must evaluate the effects of the five flavors and five fluids. Then he will correlate what he knows about a patient's condition, based partially on these relationships and partially on other information, with the way the various organs regulate the subordinate parts of the body—the muscles, bones, and skin. He consistently employs the interactions of the five elements, which all correspondencies follow (see Figure 14), and crosschecks every factor until he arrives at the indisputable center of the illness, which is invariably the point at which Yin and Yang are out of balance.

Western doctors find this system baffling, and not a little silly from a medical standpoint. Acupuncturists use it, whether they are confronted with a cold or leprosy (both of which respond well to acupuncture). Mathematical computations form a large part of the acupuncturist's art, but they are mathematical in the Chinese sense, where the function of numbers, not their quantity, determines importance.

The young Chinese man studying to become an acupuncturist must become intimately familiar with Yin-Yang theory and the correspondencies. But even when he has mastered them he will not be ready to take up the needles in a village shop or city hospital. They are concepts easily learned and remembered by someone born into Chinese society. Before they are useful to him in alleviating human misery, the acupuncturist must become more sensitive and perceptive than any Western doctor. He must learn to find any one of over three hundred acupuncture points by touch alone and to distinguish between twelve different pulses. He must master the laws of acupuncture and the meridians.

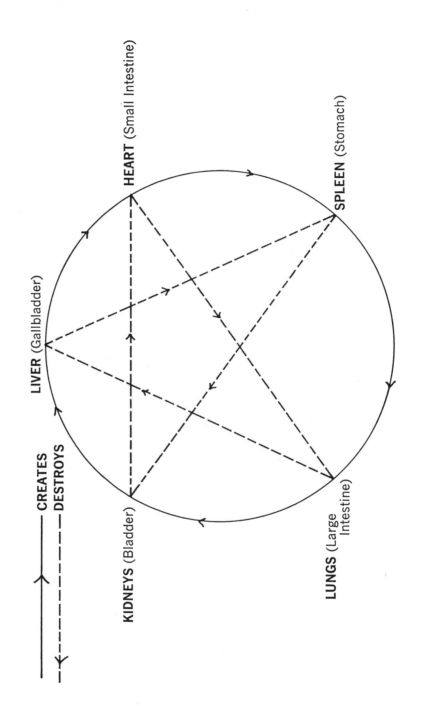

CREATES
DESTROYS

HEART (Small Intestine)

SPLEEN (Stomach)

LIVER (Gallbladder)

KIDNEYS (Bladder)

LUNGS (Large Intestine)

FIG. 14 INTERRELATIONSHIPS OF TS'ANG ORGANS AND FU VISCERA

The organs and viscera interact in exactly the same way as the Five Elements. They are capable of creating and destroying each other; that is, they can strengthen and weaken one another according to the relationships depicted in the circle above. In the practice of acupuncture, these relationships are taken into account, since any treatment of one organ will affect others.

CHAPTER V

THE ACUPUNCTURIST

*The superior doctor prevents illness; the
mediocre doctor cures imminent illness;
the inferior doctor treats actual illness.*
—Chinese Proverb

"Chinese practitioners or healers are an in-
congruous, diversified, variable, motley group of
physicians, leeches, empirics, and impostors. . . .
A large number of the sick are treated by these
classes. They are pretenders to knowledge and
skill . . . and are exploiters of the credulity of those
more ignorant and credulous than themselves.
They are shrewd, stupid, wicked exploiters of
human life. . . . Probably eighty percent of the
medical practices in China are carried out by
charlatans."

The words are those of a well-qualified Western
Physician, William R. Morse, M.D., C.M., F.A.C.S.,
LL.D. Prior to the Communist revolution in 1949, Dr.
Morse served as Dean of the Medical School, Head of
the Department of Anatomy, and Associate in Surgery
at the College of Medicine, West China Union University. British by birth, Dr. Morse chose to live and work
in China, bringing the miracle of modern medicine, as
he saw it, to the backward Chinese.

Morse based his opinion of Chinese doctors on personal observations made in the teeming city streets of Chengtu, in Szechuan province, where West China Union University was located. He lived among the Chinese people during one of the worst periods in their history, a time torn by the brutality of a government supposedly constructed to bring democracy to the masses—the same Kuomintang under Chiang Kai-shek that established concentration camps—and the steadily growing seed of violent revolution.

For eight centuries a rigid system of examinations had been used to accredit doctors. Under the Kuomintang it collapsed. In an effort to bring Chinese society to a level equal with the West's, Chiang Kai-shek had obliterated the classical learning methods and oral examinations by scholars. Chiang's motives were good; the examinations, which covered everything from civil service jobs to university professorships, made it impossible for the ninety percent of the people who were illiterate to rise in life. But for the practice of medicine, the step proved disastrous. It removed the only sanction for doctors that China had. Anyone who could afford a set of needles might call himself a doctor of acupuncture.

Hundreds of street-corner quacks appeared. From them Morse gathered his impressions of Chinese physicians and passed them on to a world hungry for news of China, much as the world is now. His book published in 1934, called *Chinese Medicine,* carried the authority of his position and eminence as a doctor. And it was nearly the only book of its kind in English written during the first half of the twentieth century.

Dr. Morse was a man with a scholarly bent. He explored the subject of Chinese medicine in great depth and careful detail, but with obvious prejudice against any form of medicine other than his own. For a man who must have come into almost daily contact with

Chinese physicians, his description of an acupuncturist
—the *only* one he gives—is remarkable.

". . . I was attracted by a large crowd in the mar-
ket place surrounding a Chinese surgeon (?) who
was *executing* the art of surgery by means of
needles in the operation of acupuncture. The operator was standing in a small square formed by
four benches with no backs; on these benches sat
the patients, and the dense crowd pressed in
closely to watch, and listen to him. That man was
no mean orator of the patent medicine class and
he had a forceful personality. He traded on human
curiosity, credulity, faith, and won—a misguided
genius. . . . His expertness was remarkable and
his patients many. He was dressed in a long gown
which had been originally blue, but which had become glistening smooth and shiny and variegated
through varying degrees of accumulated droplets
of soup and grease dropped while inhaling his
food. There had been many a slip betwixt bowl
and lip.

"On his feet were cloth-soled shoes which had
incorporated into their texture material of the
general color and consistency of mud. This . . .
material was accumulated from passing through
the wet streets where dogs, chickens, pigs, ducks,
and children, equally careful in their toilet, had
contributed their quotas. His shoes were an ento-
mologist's paradise of uncountable specimens. . . .
On the ground before him were spread four large
charts. These charts explained something of his
supposed theory and were attractive because of
their heritage of four thousand years. They very
deeply impressed his audience. These charts
showed the places which talented ancients had
indicated as safe for the needles' entrance. . . .

"Some of the needles were inserted before I
arrived, some I saw inserted. One insertion was
rather striking and gruesome. The needle entered

the nose until it reached, I would think from its direction, the ethmoid plate [bone at the base of the nose—Author] and then was struck a considerable blow, I presume piercing . . . the brain!

". . . No place seemed sacred or free from the ubiquitous needle. The operator's procedures for sterilization varied. No application was made to the skin. He 'cleaned' the needle with his thumb nail, rubbed it through his hair, or rubbed it off on his gown or the sole of his shoe, or all of these, then lubricated the needle with spittle and drove it home!"

Not a very pretty picture, to say the least. And not a very fair one. It led Dr. Morse to form this conclusion about Chinese medicine:

"At the present time, in actual practice, the majority if not all of their healing practices consist of a medley of philosophy, religion, superstition, magic, alchemy, astrology, divination, sorcery, demonology and quackery."

In the years Dr. Morse worked at West China Union University it seemed that the West and Western medicine would forever maintain a foothold in China. The Communist revolution changed that assumption, and as the missionaries, teachers, physicians, businessmen, and soldiers of foreign nations left the Chinese mainland, the government resumed control over the practice of medicine and other professions. Yet even before these events Dr. Morse's view had little basis in truth. In 1934 there were 380,000 traditional physicians in China and only a handful of Western doctors. Dr. Morse himself gave the reason:

"The Chinese people have a high grade of culture and civilization. They are intelligent, clever people. Four hundred million of Chinese cannot be continually fooled. Some scores of several hundreds of millions cannot be hoodwinked for thirty of forty centuries. . . . There is no doubt that many physicians have been successful in their ministrations. Whether their premises were erroneous or not, many of their patients got well. It may be that our eyes are [unable to see] some of their skill, it might be that we are too superior in our own conceits to recognize all the ability that we should in others!"

It is indeed difficult to believe that the most civilized nation on earth, except in terms of scientific technology, would allow the kind of medicine that Dr. Morse observed to exist for thousands of years. It did not. The doctor ignored certain facts in his writings, such as that the people continued to support traditional medicine even after Western techniques became available, and that only a small percentage of acupuncturists were quacks. Today, fully forty percent of the hospitals, clinics, and medical schools in China practice and teach only traditional Chinese medicine. Thirty percent of all medical students study acupuncture exclusively, and one-third of the training of all other medical students is in the traditional healing arts.

Many Western physicians refuse to take Chinese medicine seriously. They choose instead to view acupuncture as a mystic art, illogical though that attitude might be in the face of the success traditional medicine has in curing illness.

In placing acupuncture alongside sorcery, alchemy, and divination, Western physicians use as their evidence the status of Chinese medicine in the twenty years just before the Communist revolution. They forget, or ignore, China's many outstanding achievements in medicine throughout history. The first medical school in China, and probably in the world, was established by an emperor's edict in the seventh century

A.D., during the Tang dynasty. Called the Imperial Institute of Physicians, the college trained 350 students at a time in herb medicine, acupuncture, and surgery (which then consisted of the treatment of fractures, skin diseases, and wounds). Tang emperors also organized the nation's doctors into the *T'ai I Hsu,* the Grand Medical Service. For the first time in any country, the state regulated medical practice and set up professional standards. Prospective doctors underwent rigorous examinations and strict laws prohibited the practice of medicine without a license. Written studies that survive from that era deal with leprosy, smallpox, measles, dysentery, cholera, dropsy, beriberi, rickets, goiter and tuberculosis, among other diseases.

The examination method China used to qualify physicians had two parts. The first was a day-long oral scrutiny of a student's knowledge by his professors. Future doctors were questioned on their familiarity with the principles of acupuncture, diagnostic techniques, and the classic texts. The scholarly doctors required near-perfection in the students' answers; a single error often meant failure.

On the second day, if the student had passed the oral examination, he would demonstrate his prowess with the silver and gold needles of acupuncture. In the testing room, he would stand opposite a life-size wooden statue of a man. The statue was covered with wax and filled with water. At the 365 acupuncture points on the body, tiny holes had been punched through the wood. There were no markings on the figure and the holes were invisible under the wax. One of the examiners would pose a situation to the student: a patient had appeared at the young doctor's shop complaining of certain symptoms. Observation and the medical correspondencies had revealed that the patient's kidneys were weak in Yang, and pulse diagnosis had confirmed the nature of the problem. The patient was born in Northern China, had a wife, two sons, and a daughter. He had arrived at the shop on a sunlit spring morning. Where, the professor asked the student, would he place the needles?

The student would name a point on one of the body's meridians, or perhaps two or three points. If he specified the correct location, the professor would invite him to demonstrate how to insert the needles, substituting the wooden statue for the patient. The student would choose from among the nine kinds of needles, find the point on the statue, and push the needle through the coating of wax, using the proper technique. If he was right, water streamed from the opening. If he was wrong, he never became an acupuncturist. Professor and student repeated the scenario many times before the examination ended.

Years of study went into the student's ability to answer the professors' questions, choose the proper acupuncture points, find the exact spots on the wooden figure, and insert the needles correctly. Examiners demanded perfection with the wooden statue because errors in the practice of acupuncture can prove costly to the patient, much more so than mistakes in Western medicine.

The ingenious wax-coated manikin dates back to the Sung dynasty. In 1027 A.D. Emperor Jen Tsung ordered Wang Wei I, a noted acupuncturist and sculptor, to cast two hollow bronze figures with all the acupuncture points marked by their names and small holes. Filled with water and covered with wax, the figurines could be used to train as well as test students. Exact replicas of the statues, or *T'ung Jen, the Men of Bronze,* are still used to teach medical students the locations of the points. With no more than a dozen exceptions, the spots marked by hoes on modern *T'ung Jen* are the same as those on the bronze originals.

Disease has changed little since the eleventh century—the causes of disease not at all—and the points of acupuncture discovered in ancient times are as useful as they ever were.

Modern Chinese medical instructors have found that teaching acupuncture with wooden statues has a drawback. It does little to instill confidence in the student that his technique will be as effective on people as it is on the lifeless dolls. During Chiang Kai-shek's reign, when the government extolled Western medicine and quacks injured thousands with their untrained use of acupuncture, the people began to doubt the worth of traditional medicine. They often used an ancient proverb to express their feelings. It said: "A clever physician will never treat himself."

When the Communists seized power, they found a way to conquer the growing prejudice against acupuncture and at the same time build medical students' confidence. Acupuncture students began practicing with the needles where they were most likely to use them correctly: on themselves. A graduate from a modern acupuncture school will have pricked himself at least ten thousand times, constantly refining his skill and touch until no question remains about his ability. Western doctors, on the other hand, consider treating themselves, and in some instances their families, a breach of ethics!

Acupuncturists also have a rather unusual way of demonstrating their confidence and skill to any patients who show skepticism. They will simply pick up the longest needle in their case and thrust it into an arm or leg, smiling as they remove it and point to the spot. They will then invite the patient to examine the skin and find any evidence that a needle has just been jabbed into it. The patient will be unable to do so, even though some of the needles of acupuncture are five inches long.

The physician does not hope to prove that acupuncture works by sticking himself, only that it is painless. His demonstration helps overcome the basic human fear that sharp objects forced into the body will inflict pain. With rare exceptions—and those purposeful—acupuncture does not hurt. Other than when they replace general or local anesthetics in surgical operations, and in a few special applications, acupuncture needles do not normally pierce nerves. They are twirled or pushed into the meridians, the channels of Ch'i beneath the skin that correspond to the twelve organs and viscera.

These meridians, or ducts, carry the force of life through the body in a specific order that parallels the vital organs and relates to the time of day. The time of day is important because of the influence nature exerts on the ebb and flow of Yin and Yang. Just as the organs and viscera are divided into Yin and Yang, so are the meridians. The *Ts'ang,* or Yin, organs—liver, heart, spleen, lungs, and kidneys—have corresponding meridians, as do the *Fu,* or Yang, viscera—the gallbladder, small intestine, stomach, large intestine, and bladder. Added to these are the meridians of the Triple Warmer (Yang) and the Gate of Life (Yin).

In the *Nei Ching,* Emperor Huang Ti's minister, *Chi Po,* says that the meridians "lie deeply hidden within the muscles." At 365 points on the body, the meridians surface to just below the skin, which is where the acupuncturist can reach them with his needles. Each of the points is one-tenth of an inch in diameter, and some of them are that close to important blood vessels and nerves. A slip, ever so slight, and the acupuncturist can injure a patient seriously or cause permanent nerve damage—a good reason not to allow anyone but a qualified professional to puncture your skin with his slim needles. Chinese acupuncturists believe that even without hitting an artery or nerve, needles placed improperly can cause great harm by upsetting the balance of Yin and Yang more than illness already has. In extreme cases, such as when Yang so overpowers Yin that the patient is near death, the mistaken needling can kill.

The belief that illness deep in the body can be treated externally is not entirely foreign to Western medicine. In acupuncture the belief is based on the concept that diseased organs produce subtle symptoms on the skin, conveyed there by the meridians. Modern biology provides a rational theory for the existence of the channels.

In its very early development, the human embryo is composed of a few simply constructed cells which will divide many times; then the genetic code within them dictates what parts of the body they will give rise to. The early cells have three parts, the ectoderm, mesoderm, and endoderm. The ectoderm, or outer covering, will specialize into the skin and hair. The endoderm, or center of the cell, will develop into the internal organs. The middle section, or mesoderm, will yield the parts of the body between the organs and skin, such as the bones, muscles, and blood vessels. Throughout the development of the human embryo, these three parts of the original cells are intimately connected. When the completely formed human being emerges from its mother's womb, the connections are gone from view, at least to the naked eye. The meridians of acupuncture represent the connections that were present between the various portions of the cells before they became parts of the human being. In another, more scientific sense, the acupuncturist treats the internal organs by pricking the points on the skin that were once vitally associated with them.

Acting not on this premise, but on their own observations, nineteenth-century Western doctors noticed that in some illnesses originating from internal organs, symptoms showed up on the skin. The skin areas that corresponded to different illnesses never varied, and the most frequent symptom was pain.

In 1893 Sir Henry Head, a British nerve specialist, noticed that some patients suffering from diseased gallbladders and kidneys felt pain in parts of the body far from the stricken organs. The pain was external, on the surface of the skin, and a specific disease always resulted in pain at the same place. He wrote an article on his discovery, categorizing the skin areas affected by different illnesses and outlining the diagnostic possibilities of his discovery. The skin areas came to be known as "Head's zones," and are now a part of basic Western medical training.

Soon doctors found that "Head's zones" were useful in treatment as well as diagnosis. Massage and heat therapy on the portions of the skin that Head designated were found to relieve painful kidney and gallbladder attacks with great success. For Western doctors in this century, Sir Henry's research opened a completely new field of treatment for serious illnesses.

German doctors were the first to see the possibilities of the British neurologist's discovery. They developed a procedure called *Heilanasthesie,* or "therapeutic anesthesia." They deadened areas of the skin to relieve pain in the internal organs, a direct parallel to acupuncture. In the United States, physicians took the German procedure and added the intravenous use of chemical anesthetics, which produced similar results. Both the European and American practices stemmed from Head's research; both used the zones he first defined. No evidence exists that Sir Henry was familiar with, or even knew of, acupuncture, but the areas of the skin he linked with the gallbladder and kidneys are the same as those used by acupuncturists to treat the same organs.

To their amazement, Western doctors found that local anesthetics injected at Head's zones not only relieved pain, but in many cases aided in curing the disease. In one of the many accidents that Western medicine seems to rely upon for creating new techniques, a doctor working under a grant from a German industrial concern discovered the principle of the meridians by mistake. He was doing research on migraine headaches, which often fail to respond to Western treatment. One of his patients had terrible attacks that nothing seemed to help. The doctor decided to inject Novocain, the local anesthetic popular in dentistry, into the patient's bloodstream. As he administered the drug, his syringe slipped and the needle went in next to the vein, rather than inside it. When he looked up at the patient to apologize for his error, the doctor was told, to his amazement, that his patient's migraine headache had disappeared completely.

Had an acupuncturist been watching the German doctor's blunder and resulting cure, he would merely have nodded his head knowingly. The doctor had hit the acupuncture point for relieving severe headaches, nothing more. The Novocain itself had done nothing. The doctor's needle struck the proper place on the proper meridian and the patient's Yin and Yang, obviously far out of proportion to cause so painful a headache, quickly returned to equilibrium.

The acupuncturist sees no miracle in being able to cure serious illness by treating it at the skin, nor does he come upon cures accidentally. The system of meridians and points is as orderly and exact as that of the correspondencies, and relates to nature just as intimately. It begins, as does most Chinese thought, with the theory of Yin and Yang.

CHAPTER VI

THE MERIDIANS OF CH'I

*When the members work joyfully the
head rises grandly and the duties of all
the offices are fully discharged. When
the head is intelligent the members are
good, and all affairs will be happily performed.*

—Emperor Shen Nung
(c. 2225 B.C.)

TO BRING the body into focus as a vehicle of Yin and
Yang, the ancient Chinese doctors examined the dual
forces closely. They knew that Yin and Yang never
exist alone, and that this primary principle would remain true in the human anatomy. Through experience
they found that the body's functions could be divided
into three distinct areas, and that the diagnosis and
treatment of illness must take them into consideration.

Each section of the body must have one Yin and one
Yang quality associated with it according to the basic
principle. They called the six resulting subdivisions of
the dual forces the Greater Yang, Lesser Yang, and
Sunlight Yang, and the Greater Yin, Lesser Yin and
Absolute Yin. Each of the six encompasses two meridians and serves as an aid to the acupuncturist when he
decides whether an illness is Yin or Yang and what
type of treatment is necessary.

94

SECTION OF BODY:	MERIDIAN:	ORGAN:
{ SUNLIGHT YANG	{ ARM SUNLIGHT YANG –	LARGE-INTESTINE
	LEG SUNLIGHT YANG –	STOMACH
{ GREATER YIN	{ ARM GREATER YIN ——	LUNGS
	LEG GREATER YIN ——	SPLEEN
{ LESSER YANG	{ ARM LESSER YANG ——	TRIPLE WARMER
	LEG LESSER YANG ——	GALL-BLADDER
{ ABSOLUTE YIN	{ ARM ABSOLUTE YIN —	CIRCULATION-SEX
	LEG ABSOLUTE YIN —	LIVER
{ GREATER YANG	{ ARM GREATER YANG —	SMALL INTESTINE
	LEG GREATER YANG —	BLADDER
{ LESSER YIN	{ ARM LESSER YIN ——	HEART
	LEG LESSER YIN ——	KIDNEYS

(Gate of Life)

FIG. 15 SECTIONS OF BODY, MERIDIANS, AND ORGANS

In order to divide the body into parts useful in treating illnesses, the Chinese found divisions of Yin and Yang and related them to the organs and meridians. Each of the three body sections has some Yin and some Yang, in varying proportions. Knowing these proportions aids the acupuncturist in finding a Yin-Yang imbalance.

One part of the body contains the Absolute Yin and Lesser Yang (see Figure 15). The Absolute Yin covers the meridians of the circulation-sex organ (Gate of Life) and the liver. The circulation-sex meridian runs along the arm from the tip of the middle finger to the chest. Thus it is an "arm" meridian, and classified in acupuncture practice as the Arm Absolute Yin meridian (see Figure 16). The liver meridian extends from the end of the big toe, along the leg, and up into the center of the torso. It is a "leg" channel, referred to in practice as the Leg Absolute Yin meridian (see Figure 17).

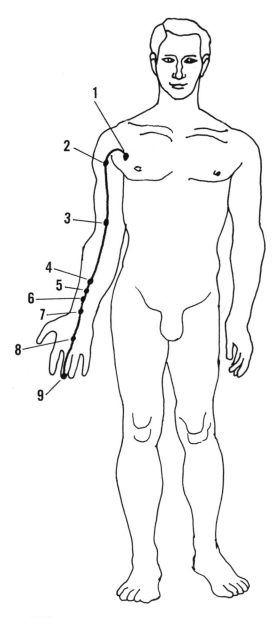

FIG. 16 CIRCULATION—SEX MERIDIAN

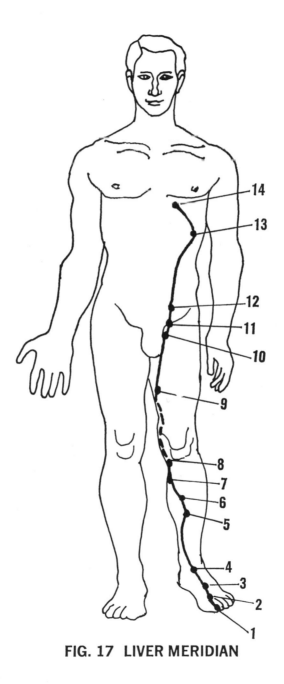

FIG. 17 LIVER MERIDIAN

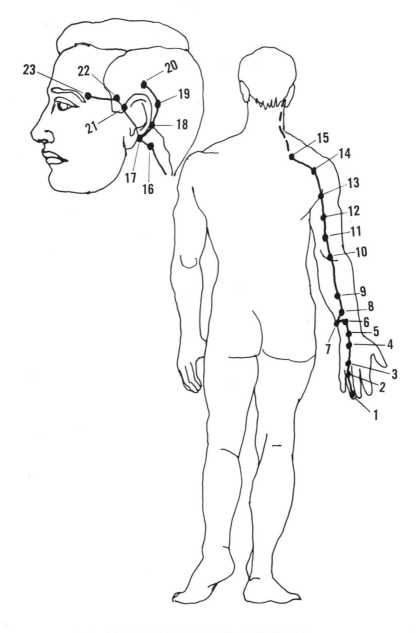

FIG. 18 TRIPLE WARMER MERIDIAN

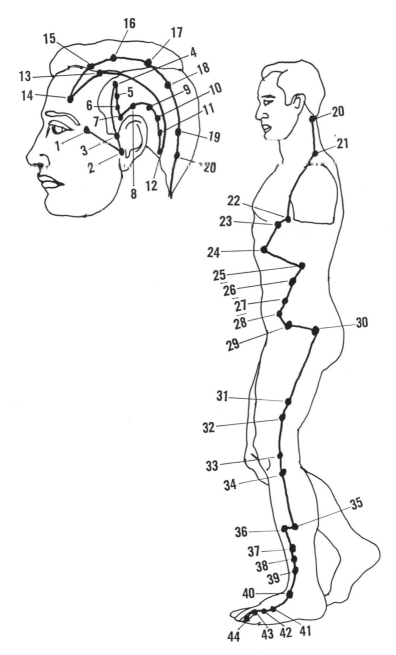

FIG. 19 GALL BLADDER MERIDIAN

(All the meridians are paired, with duplicates of the channel on each half of the body. However, both ancient and modern texts discuss only the meridians on one side or the other and refer to them singly, probably to avoid confusion. This explanation will follow that practice.)

The Lesser Yang meridians are the Triple Warmer and gallbladder. The Triple Warmer meridian starts at the hand, runs up the arm, shoulder, and neck, and ends at the corner of the eye. It is called the Arm Lesser Yang meridian (see Figure 18.) The gallbladder duct extends from the middle of the head down along the body to the bottom of the little toe, and is known as the Leg Lesser Yang meridian (see Figure 19.)

Since Yin is manifested in the earth and Yang in heaven, it would seem that the regions of the body should be divided so that the upper part is Yang, because it is nearest the sky, and the lower part Yin, because it is closest to the earth. The meridians should also parallel the concept: those in the upper section of the body should be Yang, those in the lower section Yin. In part, this is true. If a man reaches upward with both arms while his feet are firmly planted on the ground, the Yin meridians will rise from the earth, and the Yang meridians will descend from the sky. But the law that Yin and Yang must exist together ends the correlation there. For example, the meridians of the Absolute Yin do not relate to each other, but to the meridians of the Lesser Yang. The meridian of circulation-sex (Yin) corresponds to the meridian of the Triple Warmer (Yang); the meridian of the liver (Yin) stands opposite that of the gallbladder (Yang). This exactly follows the medical correspondencies, where the liver is the *Ts'ang* organ that has as its relative the gallbladder, a *Fu* viscera.

Ancient Chinese doctors found that the *Ts'ang* organs and *Fu* viscera were related in function. An imbalance in the Yin and Yang of the liver would produce an upset in the gallbladder. They discovered that treating one would exert an influence on the other, as the correspondencies suggested. The meridian system had to fit with the correspondencies of the organs for acupuncture to work. Otherwise the needles would not fully restore the Yin-Yang balance, and illness could not be cured.

In daily practice the acupuncturist uses the relationships between the organs and meridians as a diagnostic tool. Patients with liver malfunctions will often feel tenderness along the liver's meridian, the Arm Absolute Yin. If the acupuncturist presses the point on the meridian that is most nearly associated with the exact illness (in the Chinese sense of Yin and Yang imbalance), the patient will feel a sharp pain. Western medicine is familiar with the effect in heart attacks. Often a heart attack victim will feel pain shooting down his left arm, or at some points along the arm. The path of the pain corresponds precisely to the heart meridian of acupuncture.

Knowledge of the meridians far outweighs an understanding of the organs in the day-to-day practice of acupuncture. The meridians do not govern the body's functions, but they carry Ch'i, and so contribute to the living human being. Whether the ability of the meridians to convey the force of life is fanciful or real has little bearing on the effectiveness of acupuncture. The meridians are definitely connected with the organs and treating them does produce an effect on the organs they represent. Unable to reach the vital organs with his needles, the acupuncturist relies completely on the acupuncture points along the meridians to practice medicine.

Each of the organs and meridians has attached to it certain symptoms of illness that the acupuncturist looks for in his patients. He uses them as a partial guide to where the needles should be placed. But before the connection between symptoms and meridians and organs can be understood, it is important to know the paths of the channels. Four of them, the Arm Absolute Yin, Leg Absolute Yin, Arm Lesser Yang, and Leg Lesser Yang, were given above. The others are:

Arm Greater Yin (lung) meridian: begins at the second rib, runs up to the shoulder and down the arm to the end of the thumb (see Figure 20).

Leg Greater Yin (spleen) meridian: begins at the big toe, moves up along the leg, across the front of the body, and ends just above the armpit (see Figure 21).

Arm Greater Yang (small intestine) meridian: starts at the end of the little finger, extends up the arm, across the back, and up along the neck to the ear (see Figure 22).

Leg Greater Yang (bladder) meridian: begins at the nostrils, runs over the top of the head, down the neck, the side of the body, and the leg, and ends at the last joint on the big toe (see Figure 23).

Arm Sunlight Yang (large intestine) meridian: starts at the end of the index finger, extends up the arm and neck and onto the face, ending near the corner of the mouth (see Figure 24).

Leg Sunlight Yang (stomach) meridian: starts at the side of the head, runs down the back and leg to the foot and along the foot to the end of the second toe (see Figure 25).

Arm Lesser Yin (heart) meridian: starts at the top end of the armpit, extends down the arm and hand to the end of the little finger (see Figure 26).

Leg Lesser Yin (kidney) meridian: begins underneath the foot at the middle of the sole, runs up

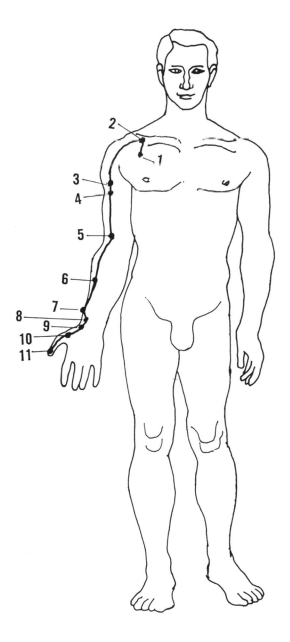

FIG. 20 LUNG MERIDIAN

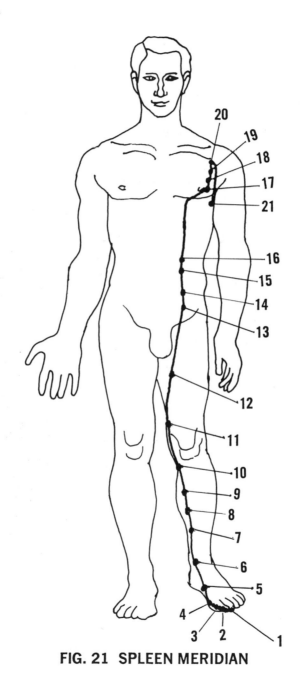

FIG. 21 SPLEEN MERIDIAN

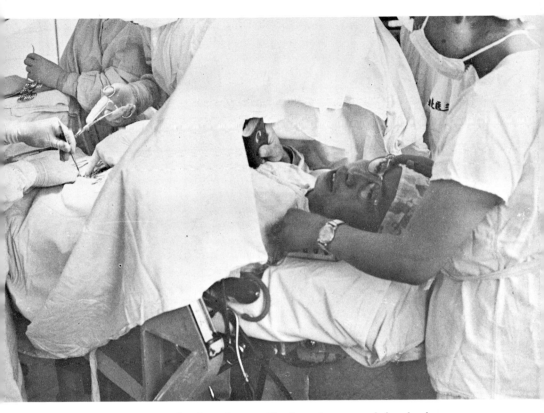

Awake, alert, and relaxed, a patient undergoes abdominal surgery with acupuncture as the only anesthesia. As the surgeons delve into his body (left) a nurse regulates the tiny electric charge introduced into the patient's nervous system via needles in his shoulder and neck (right). The process is called *electroacupuncture*. In his hand, the patient clutches a book of Chairman Mao's sayings. (Arthur W. Galston/Dispatch News Service)

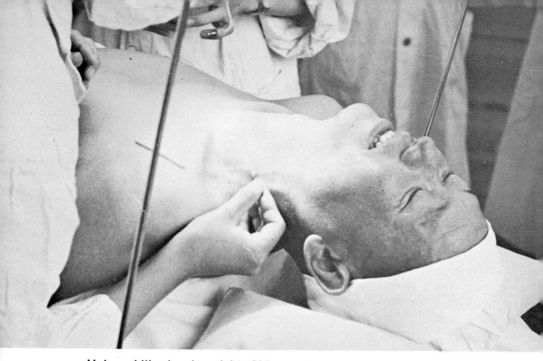

Using skills developed by Chinese doctors over four thousand years ago, a nurse inserts an acupuncture needle into a patient's neck, preparing him for major surgery. Acupuncture has served as the only form of anesthetic in more than four hundred thousand operations performed in China since 1968.

(Arthur W. Galston/Dispatch News Service)

Doctors wait while the first needle reduces the patient's ability to feel pain. The patient remains awake.

(Arthur W. Galston/Dispatch News Service)

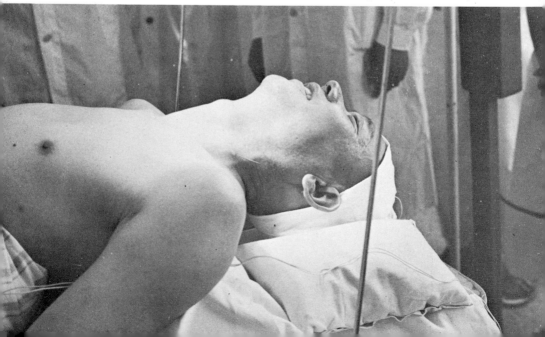

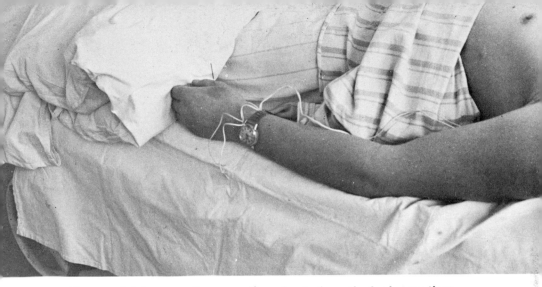

To completely erase the sensation of pain from the body, another needle is inserted into his hand.
(Arthur W. Galston/Dispatch News Service)

Nearly ready for surgery to begin, the patient waits as doctors probe his body with pins to ensure that the acupuncture has taken effect.
(Arthur W. Galston/Dispatch News Service)

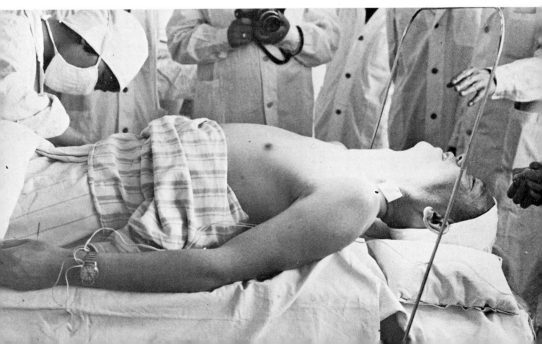

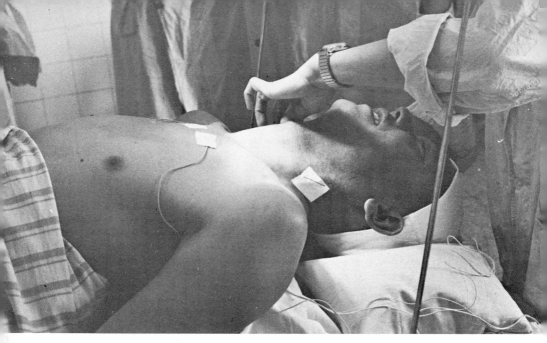

With the addition of electrodes on his chest, which will monitor his vital signs, surgery is about to begin. A sheet will be placed over the metal tubing, blocking the patient's view while the surgeons perform the operation.

(Arthur W. Galston/Dispatch News Service)

An acupuncture specialist prepares another patient for surgery. She is twirling a needle into place in his leg. The small box on the table contains the controls that enable her to regulate the flow of electricity to the needles, thus increasing or decreasing the effect of the acupuncture.

(Arthur W. Galston/Dispatch News Service)

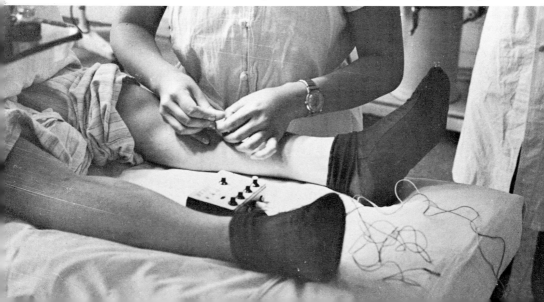

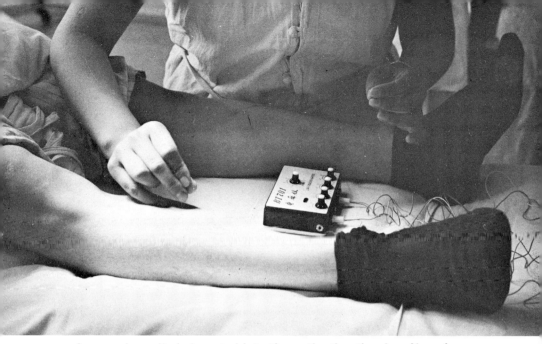

A second needle is inserted into the patient's other leg. No pain is felt when the needles pierce the skin.
(Arthur W. Galston/Dispatch News Service)

With the needles attached to the control unit, the *electro-acupuncture* and the operation can begin.
(Arthur W. Galston/Dispatch News Service)

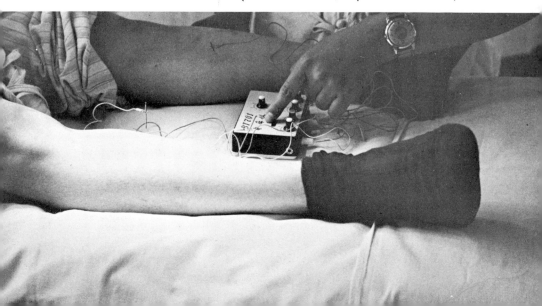

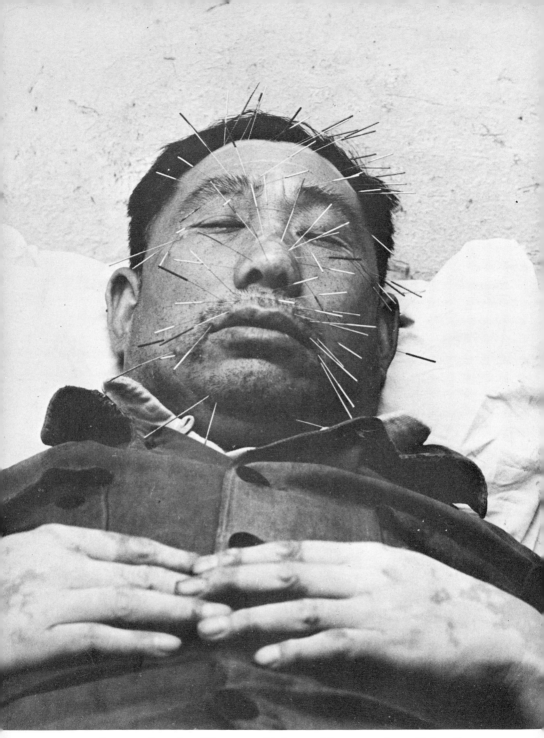

Acupuncture is still more widely used in general medicine than as an anesthetic. This man is receiving treatment for facial paralysis at a Peking hospital.

(Copyright Paolo Koch /Photo Researchers, Inc.)

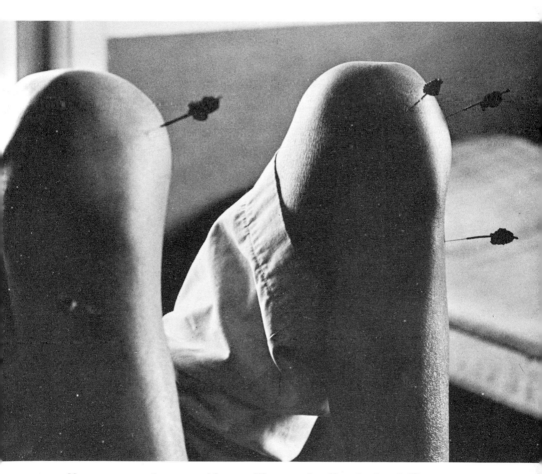

Here acupuncture combines with moxabustion to treat illness. Small piles of moxa, the leaves of the Chinese wormwood tree, are burned at the ends of the needles. Moxabustion is often used alone, with the leaves burned while they rest on the skin.

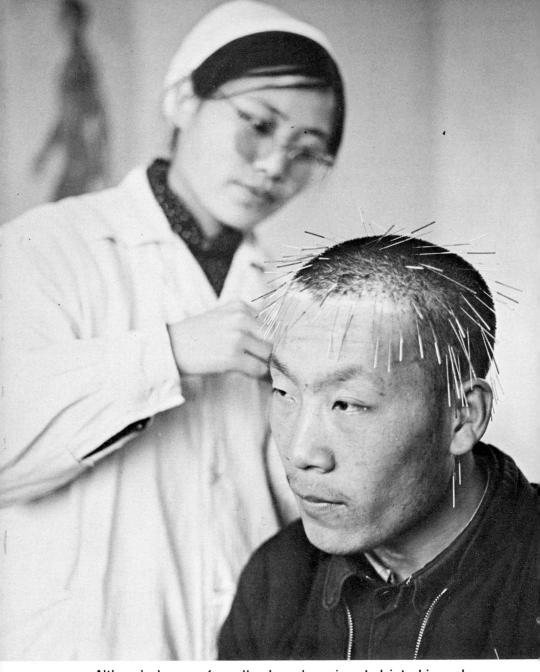

Although dozens of needles have been inserted into his scalp, this man feels no pain or other discomfort. He is being treated for migraine headaches.

(*Copyright Paolo Koch*/Photo Researchers, Inc.)

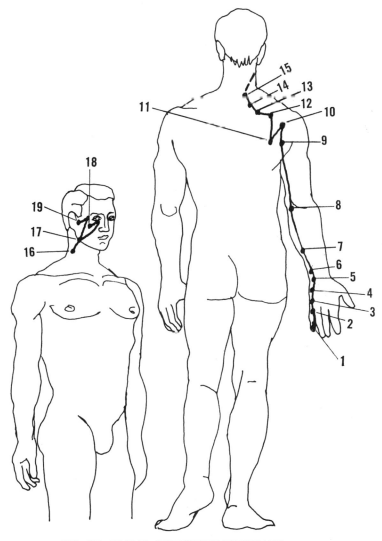

FIG. 22 SMALL INTESTINE MERIDIAN

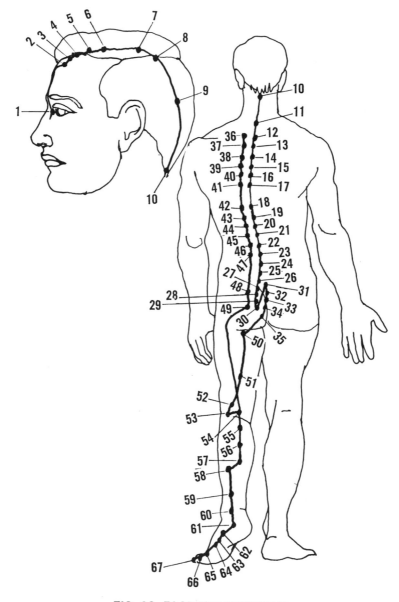

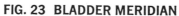

FIG. 23 BLADDER MERIDIAN

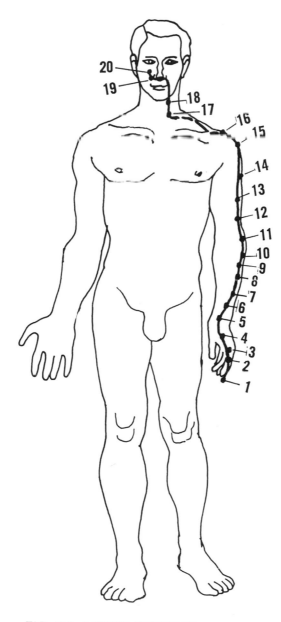

FIG. 24 LARGE INTESTINE MERIDIAN

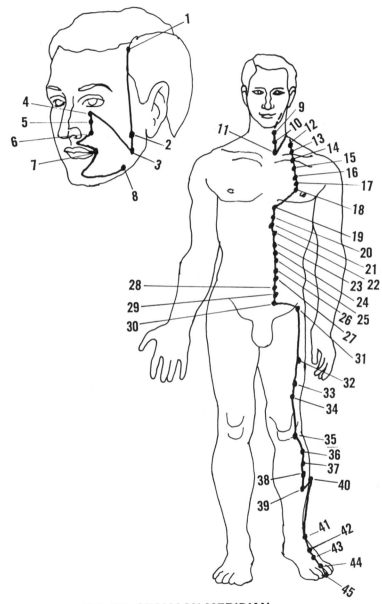

FIG. 25 STOMACH MERIDIAN

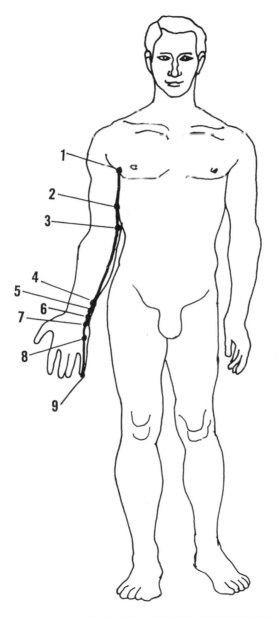

FIG. 26 HEART MERIDIAN

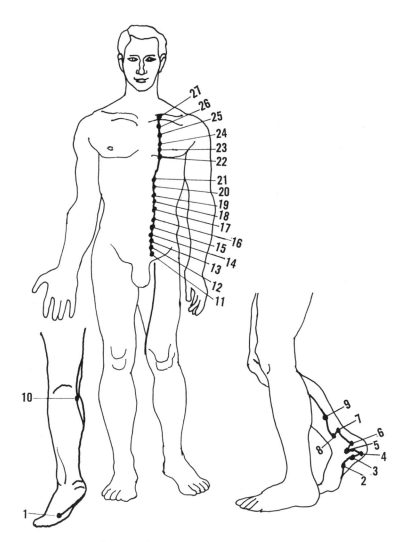

FIG. 27 KIDNEY MERIDIAN

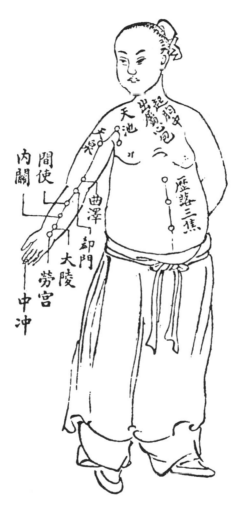

FIG. 28 THE ARM ABSOLUTE YIN (Circulation-Sex) MERIDIAN (Figs. 28-39 date back to 2600 B.C.)

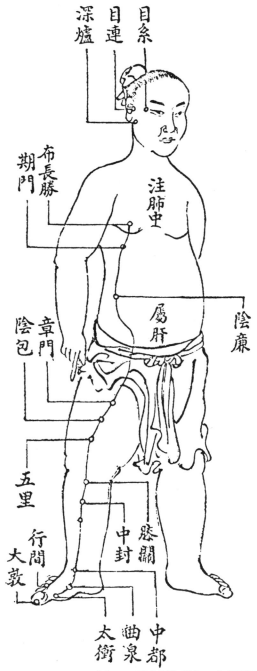

FIG. 29 THE LEG ABSOLUTE YIN (Liver) MERIDIAN

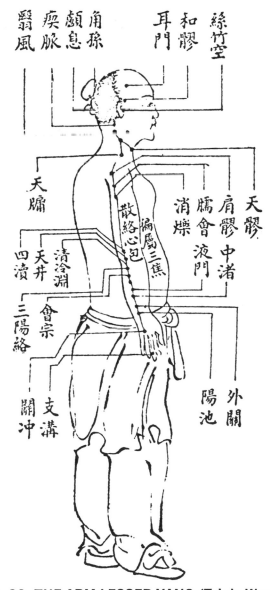

**FIG. 30 THE ARM LESSER YANG (Triple Warmer)
MERIDIAN**

the leg, along the front of the body, and ends near the top of the chest between the breasts (see Figure 27).

The paths of the meridians, like the points along them, have changed little since ancient times. The second part of the *Nei Ching*, called *Ling Shu*, deals with practical application of the concepts given in the first part, the *Su Wen*. It included drawings of the meridians that acupuncturists followed in their work. Comparison between the early illustrations (see Figures 28 to 39) and the modern charts shows little difference in the meridians. Later medical writers produced charts that combined the meridians on one human shape (see Figures 40 to 42). Many acupuncturists still use these charts in daily practice, although in the last ten years newer, easier to read reproductions have been published in China. On both the *Nei Ching* diagrams and the later composite drawings the acupuncture points are marked and named.

The relationship of the meridians to the twelve organs gives the impression that acupuncture cures any illness just by the insertion of a needle in one of the 365 specified points. The thousands of ailments that man contracts appear to boil down to just those spots along the meridians. This is untrue, and no reputable acupuncturist will claim it is so. The system is far more complex than the twelve meridians show. They are only the main meridians and the points along them are just the primary points of treatment. Two more meridians, the Governing Vessel and the Vessel of Conception, have important relationships with the body's overall well-being (the points along them are included in the 365). But that is just the beginning.

From each of the main meridians a number of

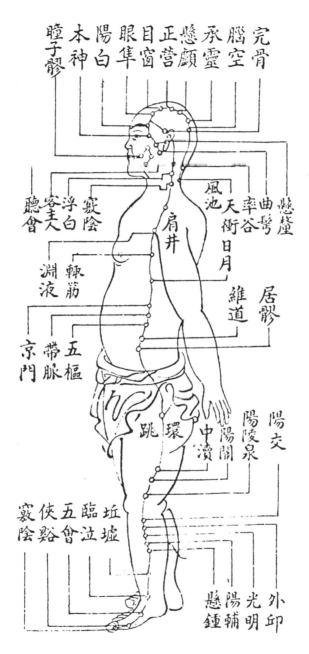

FIG. 31 THE LEG LESSER YANG (Gallbladder)
MERIDIAN

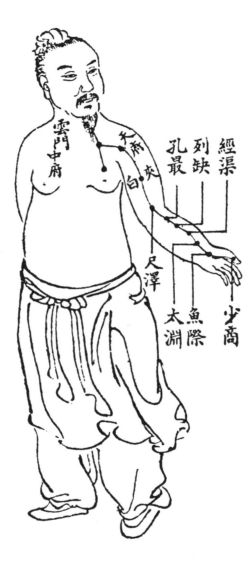

FIG. 32 THE ARM GREATER YIN (Lungs) MERIDIAN

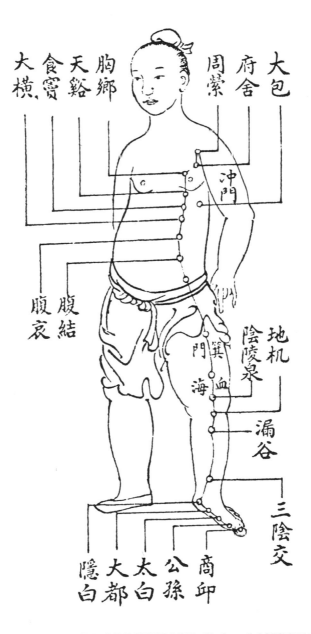

大橫
食竇
天谿
胸鄉

周榮
府舍
大包

沖門

腹哀
腹結

地机
陰陵泉

箕門
血海

漏谷

三陰交

隱白
大都
太白
公孫
商邱

FIG. 33 THE LEG GREATER YIN (Spleen) MERIDIAN

branch meridians emanate, depending on the primary meridian's length. Fifteen *Luo* channels connect the main meridians to each other. There are twelve muscle meridians and eight more that are not connected with any of the others. In all, acupuncturists use fifty-nine meridians in their work, and up to one thousand points. The number of the known points has been a basis for argument since the time of Huang Ti and *Chi Po*. Some modern acupuncturists claim that the points along the secondary meridians have no effect, while others profess to use them every time they treat a patient. No classical texts acknowledge any more than the basic 365. Even without the extra points, acupuncturists must consider all of the meridians as they interact with the organs and each other under the laws of Yin and Yang.

Symptoms correlate with specific meridians often enough for acupuncturists to form basic rules about where to look for a Yin-Yang disturbance. There are also different types of disturbances that acupuncturists must consider, due to the nature of the flow of Ch'i. Some Yin-Yang imbalances are caused by an excess or shortage of Ch'i to an organ, meaning that the force is building up inside another organ and not flowing in accordance with its flow in nature. Others are caused by too much Yin or Yang within an organ, or too little. Still others are due to a total absence of Ch'i in an organ, which might cause a collapsed lung. Any of these problems will cause sickness, and all will respond to properly used needles.

Through centuries of practice, acupuncturists have found that certain illnesses always cause the same symptoms, much as Western doctors know that the type of symptoms a disease causes are fairly consistent from person to person. This allowed acupuncturists to cate-

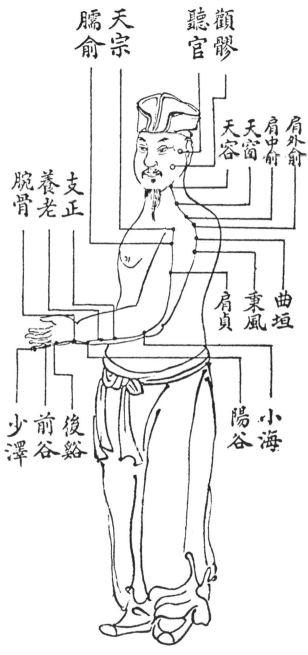

FIG. 34 THE ARM GREATER YANG (Small Intestine) MERIDIAN

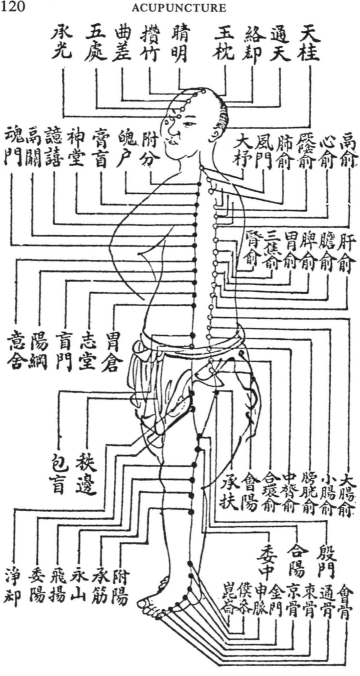

FIG. 35 THE LEG GREATER YANG (Bladder) MERIDIAN

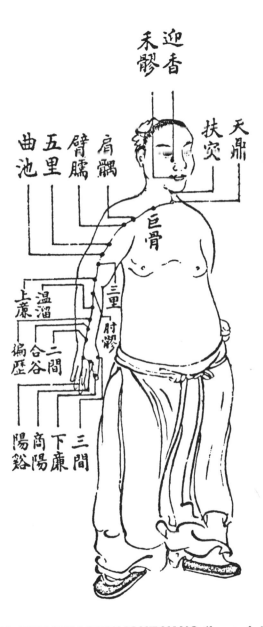

**FIG. 36 THE ARM SUNLIGHT YANG (Large Intestine)
MERIDIAN**

gorize illnesses and treatments, as long as they remembered that the human body could be inconstant. Few acupuncturists will apply the needles without first exploring every possibility of where a Yin-Yang balance might have been changed. They are cautious because they know how destructive the needles can be if used improperly.

After eight years of research, the Peking School of Chinese Medicine found that enough symptoms, meridians, organs, and illnesses could be categorized to make a listing of them useful to acupuncturists. The People's Hygiene Publishing House issued the compilation in 1960. It included the points to be used in treating various illnesses, as well as both ancient and modern explanations of their causes. Many, but not all, of the medical problems that can be helped by acupuncture were given. The list included influenza, mumps, laryngitis, tracheitis, hysteria, asthma, bronchitis, pneumonia, emphysema, pleurisy, gastritis, poor digestion, fevers, dysentery, diarrhoea, colitis, cholera, vomiting, hiccoughs, peptic ulcers, abdominal pains and distension, intestinal inflammations and spasms, and constipation.

It also listed jaundice, abdominal swellings, varicose veins, oedema, facial spasms, convulsions, insomnia, nervous tension, headaches, migraines, vertigo, syncope, meningism, neuralgia, rheumatism, lumbago, sciatica, numbness in various places on the body, paralysis, night sweats, hemorrhoids, nephritis, cystitis, retention of urine and lack of control, impotence, frigidity, lack of sexual desire, nymphomania, eczema, acne, gingivitis and similar dental problems, tonsilitis, stuttering, glaucoma, conjunctivitis, cataracts, hay fever, sinusitis, nasal polyps, beriberi, and rectal prolapse.

Among the diseases and ailments peculiar to women,

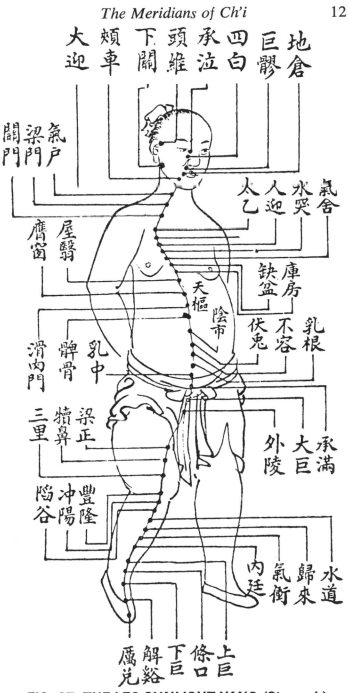

FIG. 37 THE LEG SUNLIGHT YANG (Stomach) MERIDIAN

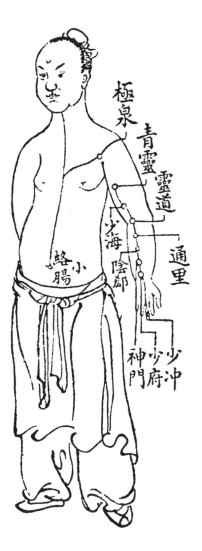

極泉

青靈

靈道

通里

少海

陰郄

絡

小腸

神門

少府

少冲

FIG. 38 THE ARM LESSER YIN (Heart) MERIDIAN

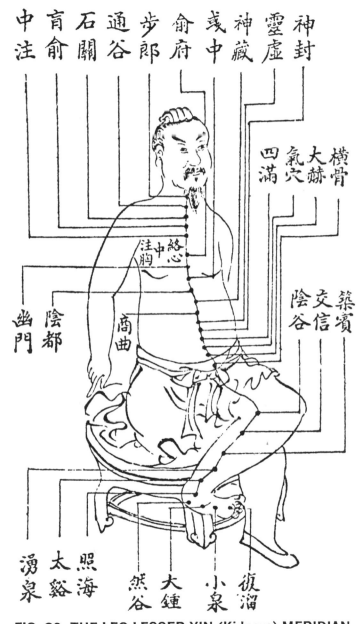

FIG. 39 THE LEG LESSER YIN (Kidneys) MERIDIAN

the report listed acupuncture treatments for irregular menstruation, sterility, excess vaginal discharge, fibroids, nausea and vomiting during pregnancy, postnatal spasms, prolonged labor, retained placenta, and insufficient production of milk.

A section of the listing was devoted to diseases of children, both emotional and physical, and hundreds of common ailments not mentioned here. It did not cover the use of acupuncture as an anesthetic, or in combination with Western techniques or other traditional healing arts.

The medical school's list was not a publicity brochure. It was issued to acupuncturists and other Chinese doctors for use as a medical reference book in their professions. Every illness that found its way into the book had been proven responsive to acupuncture alone, and doctors could use it with confidence. As a guide to verified successes with the needles, acupuncturists use the list to check their own diagnoses. But it does not replace the ancient guidelines and theories, and many practitioners will disregard the government list in favor of what experience and observation of patients teaches them.

Acupuncturists handed down the symptoms and the organs they led to from generation to generation. They found and passed on, for example, that coughing, shortness of breath, thirst, disquiet, colds, pains and aches in the chest, chills, sneezing, excess phlegm, and difficulty in breathing pointed to an imbalance in the channel of the lungs, the Arm Greater Yin meridian.

The Yin influence in the lungs is at its maximum in relation to the Yang influence, as the name Greater Yin suggests. Greater Yin meridians have a larger proportion of Yin than Yang at all times, if the body is healthy. Greater Yang meridians have more Yang than Yin. In the Sunlight Yang and Absolute Yin meridians (and organs), Yin and Yang are equal. Combined with

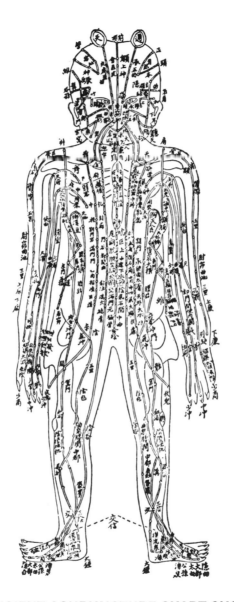

**FIG. 40 ANCIENT ACUPUNCTURE CHART SHOWING
THE MERIDIANS AND POINTS**

This illustration and the following two (Figs. 41 and 42)
are approximately 2,500 years old.

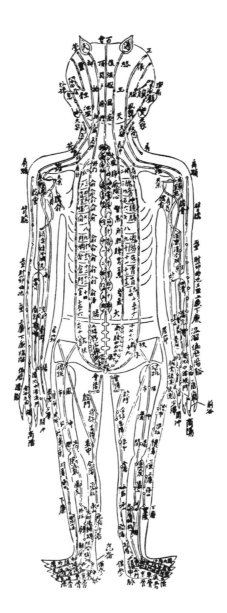

FIG. 41 ANCIENT ACUPUNCTURE CHART, rear view.

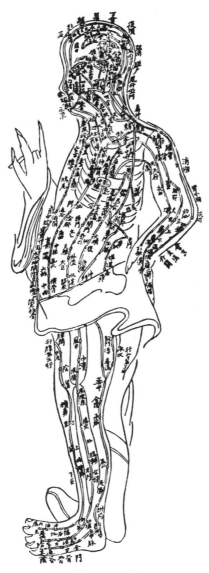

FIG. 42 SIDE VIEW OF MERIDIANS

Acupuncture Points Are Marked by Circles and Names in Chinese

the fact that symptoms are divided into those that are Yin and those that are Yang, the Yin-Yang composition of the meridians helps the acupuncturist decide what kind of imbalance has occurred.

In the Arm Greater Yin meridian, chills, a Yin symptom, indicate that the Yin influence is too strong. With his needles the acupuncturist will either increase the activity of the Yang, or decrease the Yin. Either will stop the chills, but only if they are not a symptom of another, more complex illness that originates in an organ other than the lungs. The acupuncturist will choose whether to change the Yin or Yang based on the season, weather, and time of day. When Yang is more prominent in nature, Yang in the body is easier to stimulate than Yin, and a cure will be more assured by using the needles to treat it. The same holds true for Yin when it is more prevalent in nature than Yang.

Along with the Arm Greater Yin meridian, the other main channels of Ch'i have symptoms ascribed to them. An imbalance in the meridian of the large intestine (Arm Sunlight Yang) will produce toothaches, swellings in the throat and neck, pain in the shoulder and upper arm, loss of finger dexterity, nasal discharges, constipation, and dizziness.

Disturbances in the Yin-Yang balance in the stomach meridian (Leg Sunlight Yang) may result in headaches, chills, flatulence, distended abdomen, weak legs, hunger, or feverishness.

Symptoms related to the meridian of the spleen (Leg Greater Yin) may include nausea, stomach pains, hiccoughs, indigestion, insomnia, a craving for sweet-tasting foods, fatigue during the day, diarrhoea, and a general feeling or illness.

A loss of Yin-Yang equilibrium in the small intestine meridian (Arm Greater Yang) may cause deafness, yellow eyes, pain in the elbow, pain in the neck, or swelling in the face.

The heart meridian (Arm Lesser Yin) will at times produce thirst, dryness in the mouth and throat, heaviness in the chest, pain or cold in the left arm, or a fever when Yin and Yang are out of balance.

Symptoms that stem from the bladder meridian (Leg Greater Yang) are painful eyes, piles, tearing, stiff toes, pains at joints, and headaches.

The kidney meridian (Leg Lesser Yin) will require acupuncture when the forehead or cheeks are dark, there is shortness of breath, loss of appetite, loss of vision, a feeling of fear, pain in the heart, unusual fatigue, impatience, abnormal amounts of energy, or dark-colored urine.

The meridian of the Gate of Life (Arm Absolute Yin) may have an imbalance of Yin or Yang when the armpits swell or are painful, the arms are cramped, the chest is swollen, the eyes are yellow, breath is short, the head feels heavy or aches, or there is a general sense of melancholy.

A disturbed balance of the dual forces in the Triple Warmer meridian (Arm Lesser Yang) will surface as pain in the ears, deafness, shoulder and arm pains, an all-over feeling of cold, or pain in the temples.

Gallbladder (Leg Lesser Yang) meridian symptoms may include eye pains, headaches, difficulty in hearing, shoulder pains, dizziness while walking, chills, or depression.

Associated with the liver meridian (Leg Absolute Yin) are pain in the liver and stomach, hernia, dryness, vomiting, shortness of temper, impulsiveness, excitability, and fatigue.

The acupuncturist combines his knowledge of the meridians and symptoms with needle techniques and with diagnostic talents that are even more startling than the use of needles to cure illness is in itself. When he finally approaches a patient with his slim, pointed carriers of health, he knows precisely where the needles will go, how deep they will be placed, how long they will be left in, and how many times they will be used.

CHAPTER VII

A CHINESE DOCTOR AND HIS PATIENT

No medicine cures old age or a withered flower.

—Chinese proverb

LONG PAST sundown on a chilly autumn night, urgent knocking arouses a village doctor from his sleep. He lights a candle, hurries to the front of his house, swings his door open wide, and lifts the flame into the darkness. A man's face, troubled and excited, flickers in from the cold.

The man bows and begs the doctor's pardon; he knows it is late. He is the servant of a wealthy farmer, and his master's wife has suddenly taken ill. The woman's condition worsens with every hour. She has a high fever and her face is waxen. The landowner has sent him to bring the doctor. Can he come immediately?

Yes, the doctor answers, and invites the servant to wait inside while he dresses and gathers what he will need for the house call. Midnight knocks on his door are common; it will take only a few moments to prepare for the short journey to the landowner's country house.

The physician looks over the acupuncture needles and herb medicines he may need to treat his patient.

133

They are in order, ready for use should his diagnosis indicate them. As he is about to leave, he picks up a small doll, perhaps eight inches long, of a nude woman. Later it will become an important aid in examining the landowner's wife.

The servant and doctor hurry through the town and out along country roads to the manor house. From a distance the well-lighted house blazes like a torch above the darkened fields. The two men are in a carriage, and at the sound of hoofbeats the landowner himself rushes from the house to the edge of the road. He welcomes the acupuncturist quickly, leaving out many of the courtesies that would normally pass between them. The doctor notices this, taking it as a sign that the farmer's wife is very ill. He suggests that they go to her at once.

In the woman's apartment, the windows are tightly shut to ward off any cold night breezes. A maidservant, who had been sponging her mistress's feverish forehead with cool water, rises and draws the curtains around her bed as she hears the men approach. They enter the room swiftly; the acupuncturist immediately strides to his patient's bedside. He sits on the chair the maidservant has left and begins questioning the landowner's wife. The questions are important, but the woman is weak, almost delirious with fever. After a few minutes the doctor stops asking them; the answers are nearly useless in diagnosing the illness.

All the while, the physician has been talking to his patient through thick curtains, unable to see her. Much later, when the house call ends, both diagnosis and treatment completed, he still will not have once looked at the landowner's wife.

Many of his patient's words have been incoherent, but the acupuncturist has learned that she is in pain, and when the pain and fever began. He puts his arm through a slit in the bed curtains and tells the woman to put her wrist in his hand. He asks the others in the room for silence. Inside the curtains, he rests the tips of his fingers on the main artery that runs down the woman's arm and into her hand, first gently, then with increasing pressure. For nearly a half-hour, the doctor concentrates on the sensations his fingers are receiving from the woman's wrist. When he has finished, he moves the chair to the other side of the patient's bed. Through another slit in the curtains he repeats the process. Again he asks for complete quiet and centers his attention on the woman's pulse.

After many more minutes pass, he pulls his hand back through the bed curtains and asks the maidservant to bring him the doll that rests on top of his needle case. He tells the landowner's wife that he needs to know exactly where she is feeling pain. He pushes the doll through the curtain, along with a crayon, and it comes back marked as close to the painful spot as the patient can manage.

The acupuncturist nods when he sees the mark on the doll. It confirms what he thinks is the problem, and makes the treatment he will prescribe more certain to cure the woman. From his silk-lined case he takes two needles, and again puts his arm through the slit in the curtains. He tells his patient to put out her arm and with his fingertips feels her forearm until he finds what he is looking for: two slightly swollen, hardened spots along the meridian that corresponds to the organ at the center of the woman's illness. These are the acupuncture points most closely associated with the ailment she has contracted. The acupuncturist twirls his needles into the two points, knowing that they will return Yin and Yang to balance in the affected organ, and alleviate the woman's suffering.

The needles are left in for the necessary time, decided by the severity of the Yin-Yang imbalance, then pulled quickly from the woman's arm. One had been inserted just above the wrist, the other near the elbow.

No sign now remains that they ever pierced the skin, but the acupuncturist must find them again with his fingertips in order to complete the treatment. He takes from his case two small piles of *moxa*, leaves of the Chinese wormwood tree, and places them on the same spots he pierced with his needles. He sets the two mounds on fire, lets them burn to the skin, then crushes the ashes into the small wounds the *moxas* make. He tells his patient to keep her arm still and assures her that, within minutes, she will begin to feel better. As he waits, she does. Her fever abates, the pain subsides, and her senses return. The doctor suggests that she avoid certain foods, and prepares an herb medicine for her to take the next morning. He says that she will feel completely well by then, but slightly weak, and that the herb remedy will help her regain her strength. He asks her to visit his shop in two weeks so that he may use his needles to stimulate her spleen, which he found a bit sluggish. She says that she will come.

The acupuncturist picks up his case and the small doll and follows the landowner out of his wife's bedroom. The farmer thanks him profusely for his service and offers him tea. The doctor declines, adding that he has been happy to help the landowner in his time of need. The crisis past, there is time for the amenities Chinese culture includes, and the two men talk at length before the doctor leaves.

Outside the house, the acupuncturist climbs aboard the carriage beside the servant who brought him. As they enter the town and approach the doctor's house, the servant remarks that he has few lanterns hung outside his door, and that therefore he must be a very fine physician. The acupuncturist smiles happily, and remarks that the ancestral spirits have been good to him. He adds that he is pleased to have treated the landowner's wife successfully. In these times, he says, the fewer lanterns the better.

It sounds like a strange comment for a doctor to make, but at the time the house call would have taken place, it was not at all unusual. During the first few centuries A.D., Chinese doctors were subject to a curious bit of discrimination, one that might be good to have around today. Every time a patient they treated died, unless he or she was very old and death was appropriate to their life-cycles, acupuncturists were forced to hang a lantern that burned throughout the night in front of their doors. Anyone passing by could see just how good—or at least how lucky—the doctor was by the number of lanterns glowing in the dark, Local citizens had an indispensable yardstick for choosing a family physician. The lantern-hanging was by imperial edict, and few, if any, acupuncturists would risk the emperor's wrath by failing to comply.

If it seems unfair to blame every patient's death on his doctor, something very few people would do today, in those times it was not. Chinese medicine by then knew much about the causes of death. Doctors had learned that life could end in many ways, for many reasons, but that, in the end, all the illnesses that result in death came back to the immutable law of the universe, the Tao. They knew that Yin and Yang control death in the body as they do life, and their medical techniques regulated Yin and Yang enough to ward off death—unless it was decreed by fate. Doctors were expected to preserve life except when, according to Tao, it was time for death.

Many changes have taken place in Chinese society since doctors hung lanterns to commemorate the deaths of their patients. The acupuncturist's house call would today be made in a much different manner, and the woman would not be shielded from his view by thick curtains. But the special status of women that made diagnosis by dolls and through slits in bed curtains necessary endured for thousands of years. For many centuries it was considered highly improper for anyone other than a woman's husband (or her maidservants) to look upon her body. Chinese women dressed in layers of clothing from head to foot, sometimes because of climate, but in the main because of propriety. This was not, as most of the West believes, due to some conception of woman as man's chattel, property to be used and disposed of at will.

Chinese women have always been held in high esteem, particularly as mothers to the nation's children. In terms of Yin and Yang, the Chinese believe that at conception Yang comes from the father and Yin from the mother. This "Yin energy," as it is called, is thought of as "primary." The "Yang energy" provided by the father is considered "secondary." Woman is like the earth, fertile and productive and life-giving. She begins the line of descendants Chinese people believe vital to the continuation of their life after death. For this reason, among others, Chinese women were for millennia protected from the rigors of life. Women have all the qualities of Yin, the dark, receptive, yielding influence. Men, by virtue of their being Yang, are the leaders, the dominant and decisive factors in family life. Chinese women were placed on pedestals, but not as useless objects of beauty to be admired and not taken seriously. The pedestals paid homage to their very special place in the scheme of the universe.

The wife in a household determines the line of descendants a family will have. She is revered not just as the mother of whatever sons and daughters she gives birth to, but also of those that will come in future generations. Coveted by the Chinese man as the embodiment of his wish for immortality, the Chinese woman has figured prominently in the development of Chinese society. She has been more honored, and protected, than her Western counterpart. Until the Communist revolution she had never been the equal of the

Chinese man, but in the sense of her importance to the survival of his spirit, she has been far superior.

Practicality, the yardstick for virtually everything done in Chinese society, caused the image of woman to take on another, less agreeable aspect. China has been an agricultural nation through nearly all its long history; the people have always depended on the land to feed and clothe them. To Chinese farmers, sons were always more valuable than daughters. While still very young, male children could work the land. In old age, parents leaned on their sons for support—daughters would marry and leave home to begin a line of descendants of their own. Except perhaps for India, no nation on earth has struggled with the depths of poverty as China has since its earliest beginnings. To destitute peasants, a female child meant another mouth to feed, another life to care for, another burden on the already overworked soil. The meager fruits of hard labor would have to be shared by more people—in the case of girl children, by people who might never return their sustenance by tilling the land.

Acupuncturists grappled with the problems of the Chinese woman's place in society as soon as the healing technique was invented. In the case of the house call described earlier, the doctor was not allowed to see his patient. Customs changed and became more liberal in later centuries, but the acupuncturist's examination of female patients was still restricted to the arms, lower legs, and face. The prohibition lasted well into this century, a burden to Chinese medicine even more hampering than the taboo on dissection of bodies. Yet acupuncturists were able to effectively diagnose and treat illnesses of all varieties in women as well as men. The special nature of their diagnostic methods made this possible, techniques that seem, to the Western physician, both useless and fanciful.

The crux of Chinese diagnosis is *sphygmology*, the

taking of the pulse. In a majority of cases it is the only diagnostic technique acupuncturists use. Nearly always it is the one that ultimately decides what is wrong, where the problem is located, and what treatment is needed.

CHAPTER VIII

THE TWELVE CHINESE PULSES

*Even the strongest medicine cannot cure
a vulgar man.*

—Chinese proverb

CHINESE DOCTORS believe that there are twelve different pulses in the body, each associated with a vital organ. They believe that they can distinguish various pulses, and from what they learn discover the seat of an illness—the Yin-Yang imbalance. Western doctors insist that there is one pulse and that it reveals only a small amount about the internal condition of the body. I asked twenty-two licensed United States physicians if it was possible, in their view, for eleven pulses to exist without their being able to find them in a patient's wrist. All who answered asked to remain anonymous, perhaps so that if future research finds them wrong, their practices will not suffer. Some of their comments, and the specialties of Western medicine the doctors practice, are enlightening:

"It simply cannot be," said a general practitioner.
"Impossible!" said a pediatrician.
"Hogwash," said another man practicing general medicine.
"The whole field of acupuncture, especially pulse diagnosis, is entirely fictitious," said a surgeon.

141

"Only in novels and communist propaganda," said
a neurosurgeon.

"I do not believe there are a dozen pulses, or that
illness could be diagnosed just from studying them
even if they did exist," said an eye, ear, nose, and
throat specialist.

"We can tell much from a patient's pulse, but not
what the Chinese claim. No, I don't believe there
are twelve pulses, just one," said a heart specialist.

Not one of the physicians admitted even the possibility that traditional Chinese doctors might be partially
right about the nature of the human pulse. The last
remark is the most peculiar, since it comes from a
doctor who uses the pulse to discover subtle facets of a
patient's condition. Trained heart specialists "read" the
pulse for many more factors than do general practitioners. From the rate, tension, and force of a pulse they
can pinpoint specific heart problems and check for
deterioration in the walls of arteries. They divide the
pulse into different parts as the acupuncturist does, but
the similarity ends there. Even the most perceptive
heart specialist detects less from the pulse than an
average traditional Chinese physician.

Acupuncturists depend on the pulses they feel to
reveal the exact nature of any illness in the body. They
believe that the pulses are never wrong. While symptoms may lead to more than one organ, or even to
none at all, the pulses are specific and undeniably
correct.

Taking the pulse in Chinese medicine differs completely from the common experience Western people
have in their doctors' offices. The acupuncturist does
not merely pick up your wrist, count the beats he feels
against a clock, and jot down the result on your medical record. A traditional Chinese physician will study
the pulses for between ten minutes and three hours. He
will attempt to discern, in each of the twelve pulses, up

to twenty-seven different qualities, all of which date back to the classic texts on medicine. Acupuncturists find, classify, and judge more than three hundred distinct characteristics in a patient's pulse, while Western doctors take note of a total of three.

The finely tuned sensitivity an acupuncturist needs to perform his craft displays itself in sphygmology, for without the pulse-taking (except in a few recently developed applications) acupuncture is not possible—at least not safely. While it is technically possible to diagnose and treat illness by acupuncture using only a patient's visible symptoms and the correspondencies, few Chinese doctors will attempt to do so. In the old style, it would put many lanterns above their doors. In addition to learning the basic medical principles, correspondencies, points, symptom correlations, effects of the environment on the body, and needle technique, the acupuncturist studies the system of pulses. His study is not merely an academic undertaking; he must use pulse diagnosis every day, on every patient he treats. With only his fingertips, he must be able to decide the exact nature of any illness, its severity, and the treatment needed to cure it.

Chinese doctors take the pulses by placing the tips of their first three fingers on the radial artery at about the same place Western doctors use. The pulse is divided into three sections and all are felt at the same time. Beginning closest to the hand, these are called the *ts'un* or inch, the *ch'ih* or bar, and the *kuan,* or cubit. The English names are direct translations of the Chinese words used in the *Nei Ching* and all modern texts. If the three pulse sections have other, more descriptive names, these have been lost over the centuries.

When a local physician prepares to take a patient's pulse in his shop, he will ask him to lie down or at least to sit quietly for ten minutes or more. He will then take one of the patient's wrists in his hand, bend it back slightly, and place the fingertips of his other hand on the pulse-taking artery. If the patient is a man, the acupuncturist will begin by feeling the pulses on his left wrist; if the patient is a woman, he will start with the right. Left is a characteristic of Yang; right is a characteristic of Yin. Normally the pulses on the left wrist of a man will reveal more about illness than those on the right. The opposite is true of a woman's pulses. Even though the sex of a patient dictates which wrist will come first, the acupuncturist studies the pulses of both sides before arriving at a complete diagnosis.

The physician's fingertips are spread apart about a half-inch, which allows him to feel the three sections of the pulse separately. Each section represents a different organ. He first lets his fingertips rest on the artery gently, then presses down harder. These are two separate portions of the procedure. In the first, the acupuncturist feels the "superficial" pulses. In the second, he takes the "deep" pulses. He receives different sensations in each position, a fact that anyone can easily confirm in this manner: first, press the tip of one index finger on the radial artery of the other wrist very lightly, feeling the beat of the pulse. After a moment, increase the pressure of the fingertip quickly without changing the position of either hand or lifting the finger. Maintain the stronger pressure for a few seconds. The sensation of the pulse will seem to disappear, then reappear, imparting a quite different sensation. After a few attempts, it will feel as though the pulses of two different people are being felt.

With each of his fingertips, the acupuncturist distinguishes pulses in the inch, bar, and cubit areas, and at the superficial and deep positions. Thus six organs are represented on each wrist. In the superficial position (gentle pressure) on the right wrist, the acupuncturist feels the pulses of the large intestine, stomach, and Triple Warmer. In the deep position (heavy pressure) the pulses of the lungs, spleen, and circulation-sex organ are felt. On the left wrist, the superficial position reveals the pulses of the small intestine, gallbladder, and bladder. The deep position is used to feel the heart, liver, and kidney pulses.

The pulses carry out the relationships of the organs and viscera and the subdivisions of Yin and Yang in the body. For example, the inch section on the right wrist yields the pulses of the lungs (deep) and large intestine (superficial). These two organs are paired with each other in the medical correspondencies. The pulse of the lungs is felt "deeply," that is, with heavy pressure. It is an internal pulse, and corresponds with a Yin

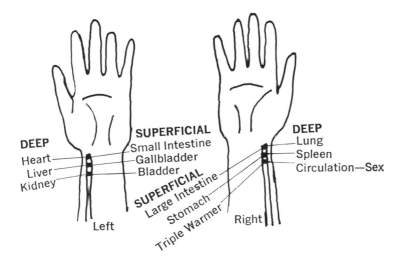

FIG. 43 PULSE DIAGNOSIS

Using their first three fingers, acupuncturists sense the pulses of the twelve internal organs on the radial artery, as shown. "Superficial" pulses are taken by applying light finger pressure. "Deep" pulses require heavy pressure. Each of the twelve pulses reveals up to twenty-seven different qualities, each an indication of a specific illness or disease.

organ. The pulse of the large intestine is felt "superficially," with gentle pressure. It is an "external" pulse, and corresponds with a Yang organ. The pulses of all six Yin, or *Ts'ang,* organs are superficial. Those of the Yang, or *Fu* viscera, are deep, following the basic characteristics of the dual forces (see Figure 43).

When an acupuncturist takes a patient's pulses, whether superficially or deeply, on the left wrist or the right, he looks for certain characteristics in each one. A healthy organ will yield a pulse with certain qualities. When the qualities differ from what is normal, illness in the organ is indicated.

In his village shop, or in one of China's modern new clinics, the acupuncturist will take his own pulse before he feels a patient's. The sensations he feels in a patient's pulses are always relative to his own. For example, any of the twelve pulses should, in a healthy person, beat four times during one respiratory cycle—one inhalation and one exhalation combined. If the acupuncturist does not know whether his pulses are normal, slow, or fast, he will not be able to judge the rates of his patient's. And because the doctor's pulses express themselves very subtly in his fingertips, any abnormality in his pulses may show up as an irregularity in those of his patient. Failure to take his own pulses into account could lead the acupuncturist into a false diagnosis and a useless or even dangerous application of the needles.

The rate of the pulse in relation to breathing is one of four basic qualities the acupuncturist senses. He checks each pulse for all of them before attempting to distinguish other characteristics. They are called *Fu, Ch'en, Ch'ih,* and *Hsu. Fu* is a superficial feeling, *Ch'en* a deep feeling. *Ch'ih* a slow feeling, and *Hsu* a rapid feeling. In describing the four basic sensations, and the hundreds of others, the special nature of the Chinese language becomes vital to the practice of medicine. Vivid word-pictures of feeling are a basic part of

Chinese. They provide the only method of conveying the different pulse qualities. The *Fu* sensation is described in the *Nei Ching* and most other medical texts as feeling like a "piece of wood floating on water." The *Ch'en* pulse is like a "stone thrown into the river." The *Ch'ih* characteristic need no vivid description, nor does the *Hsu*. The pulse is slow when it beats three or fewer times in one respiratory cycle and rapid when it reaches uin or more.

The acupuncturist compares these characteristics of each pulse to the way normal, healthy pulses act. Every pulse should flow freely, without hesitation, yet be elastic. It should be calm, but persist with a certain tension. To learn the subtle distinctions between these characteristics, an acupuncturist must study with a master sphygmologist, who will constantly check and correct his diagnosis of any ailment. The sensitivity and knowledge required to take the pulse accurately can be acquired only after years of practice.

Once the acupuncturist checks each pulse for the four basic qualities, he proceeds to the characteristics that denote specific illnesses. Opinions about some of the characteristics differ from doctor to doctor, just as the implications of various symptoms are not agreed upon by physicians in the West. But most of the pulse qualities are widely accepted and used by all acupuncturists. In any of the pulses, the acupuncturist may find that the pulse differs from being healthy in as many as a dozen ways at one time. He may feel that a pulse is buoyant, floating, feeble, slippery, tight, large, stretched, unassuming, crouched, timid, hidden, or frail. Or he might sense that it is scattering, slender, hollow, wiry, tardy, thready, ropy, overflowing, or bounding. There are many more, and each is significantly different from the others. Each implies a different illness, and all rely on the Chinese language to make them understandable. A slippery pulse will feel like stones rolling along the bottom of a smooth kettle. A hollow pulse is like an onion stalk. A hard pulse is tense, like the surface of a drum. A soft pulse is like a thread floating on water. Every pulse quality has a similar kind of description attached to it. No other language can relay exact images as easily as Chinese, for no other language is based on images as concrete.

As he takes the pulses, the acupuncturist must remember that they will differ slightly even in healthy people. Someone who is lively and energetic will have stronger, more urgent pulses than someone who is lethargic and slow. The differences do not reflect abnormalities that indicate illness. It is normal for a highly paced person to have a faster pulse than someone who is average, or slowly paced.

After he finishes taking the pulses, the acupuncturist compares the irregularities he has found with the illnesses that affect the various organs and viscera. The relationship between the pulses, illnesses, and organs is constant. A wiry pulse at the large intestine tells the acupuncturist that his patient has intestinal parasites. An elevated, hard pulse in the same spot indicates constipation. Acupuncturists make specific diagnoses based only on the pulses. Often they are more accurate than Western doctors using modern machines and laboratory equipment. In China, Europe, and the Soviet Union, acupuncturists use pulse diagnosis to pinpoint diseases Western doctors are unable to localize, and therefore unable to cure. Five hundred thousand traditional physicians in China rely on the pulses as their basic diagnostic tool. Even the decision whether or not to use acupuncture rests on the outcome of pulse diagnosis. If it indicates an illness or disease known to be unresponsive to the needles, a doctor will recommend herb remedies or, now, Western treatments.

The acupuncturist must also consider the seasons when he takes the pulses. Since the human body responds to changes in nature, so will the pulses. In spring the pulses will be slow, slippery, and gentle. They will feel like the stings of a lute. In summer the pulses will be stronger, but will fade away quietly. They will be like a sickle cutting through tall grass, or a hammer, sharp when it hits and silent as it leaves. In autumn the pulses will beat lightly and wane quickly. In winter the pulses will be deep and urgent. Pulses that do not act as they should according to the seasons indicate illness.

From the way a pulse feels compared to what is normal for the specific person and season, the acupuncturist decides whether Yin or Yang has moved out of proportion. If all the pulses are too strong, hard, or full, too much Ch'i is present in one organ or another. The acupuncturist will use his needles to move Ch'i to where it belongs. If the superficial pulses are too hard, strong, or full, too much Yang is present. If too much Yin is present, the deep pulses will be wavering, light, and hesitant. The acupuncturist tailors his treatment to return the balance to normal. Another clue to which of the dual forces is out of hand is the relative strength of the pulses in the different sections on the artery. Should the *ts'un* section (nearest the hand) be stronger than the *kuan* (farthest from the hand), Yang is overpowering Yin. The opposite means that Yin has become too powerful. Many other factors inform the acupunturist about the Yin-Yang balance in the organs. Each factor is relative to all the others, and every one is taken into account before the acupuncturist even picks up his needles.

Taking the pulse is not an archaic technique likely to pass from popularity with the introduction of Western medicine into China. The list of illnesses treatable by acupuncture published by the Peking School of Chinese Medicine in 1960 included the correct pulse diagnosis for each ailment. The pulse characteristics it contained were the same as those first described in the *Nei Ching*. All had proven useful in clinical studies performed at the college.

Traditional Chinese physicians use the pulses for more than diagnosing illness. Some acupuncturists claim they can predict the sex of a baby by studying the mother's six superficial pulses at a certain stage of the pregnancy. When she will give birth to a boy, the pulses on the left wrist will be rapid. If it is to be a girl, those on the right wrist will increase in speed. A number of pulse characteristics are said to warn of impending death, although opinions differ among acupuncturists as to their reliability.

The most remarkable talent of a master pulse diagnostician is his ability to detect illness long before it appears as noticeable symptoms. The pulses mirror even the slightest upset in an organ. The early Chinese doctors knew that the pulse depends on the flow of blood, but they believed that the flow of Ch'i through the organs and meridians directly controls the circulatory system. Western physicians know that long before an illness becomes apparent in the body, it has taken hold in one of the organs. In some instances, Western diagnostic methods can find illness before it becomes known to the patient. Early detection of tuberculosis is a well-known example. Chinese doctors believe that *every* illness shows up in the pulses before it causes overt symptoms and that pulse diagnosis reveals the symptoms months, or even years, in advance. The West scoffs at this belief, but China does not. Tens of millions of Chinese people visit acupuncturists regularly to have hidden illnesses diagnosed and treated.

The image of acupuncture as some mysterious form of magic owes much to the early diagnosis of illness by pulse-taking. It is natural for a layman told by a doctor that in three years he will develop a certain liver disease, who does contract the illness at the specified time, to think of the physician as a man with unnatural powers. If, as some acupuncturists do, the doctor also tells a patient he has never seen before what his medical history is, the impression of the acupuncturist as a magician, seer, or even sorcerer, will be even stronger. Not all acupuncturists are adept enough to read a patient's medical past or future in his pulses, but many are. The pulses reveal any residual effects of illness anywhere in the body, even scar tissue. Any malfunction in an organ, no matter how slight, will be detected by a proficient pulse-taker.

Pulse diagnosis is the most exciting possibility acupuncture presents to the world. If a future illness can be detected by nothing more than studying a patient's pulses, it can usually be stopped in its initial stages—by acupuncture or other treatment. The West is slowly awakening to what this can mean for the world's masses. Doctors in Germany and France, two of the foremost nations in medicine, who are trained in both Western and Chinese medicine use pulse diagnosis daily. If illness or disease can be detected at its earliest point, it can be treated more quickly and less expensively than when it puts the human body into a state of sickness. Widespread and expert pulse diagnosis could save thousands, if not millions, of people the expense of prolonged medical care, and prevent the permanent damage that many diseases cause. The amount of human misery and suffering that could be avoided staggers the imagination. The number of years that could be added to human life is inestimable. The reduction in cost to taxpayers who must support those unable to work would run into the billions of dollars. No measurement exists for the uplift in morale early detection of illness could bring, nor can the self-respect gained by men otherwise unable to support their families be estimated .

Detection of future illness by taking the pulse is far

from a perfected art, even though Chinese doctors have been working at it for four thousand years. Many conditions must be met before it is possible. The patient's age, physical condition, and medical history are important, as are the climate, time of year, time of day, and the acupuncturist's sensitivity and experience. But for the possibilities it presents, much too little research into the subject is being done. In some nations, such as the United States, pulse diagnosis is almost completely unknown, and no work has been started toward even evaluating its potential. A medical technique that could fulfill the wish of every dedicated physician, and certainly every patient—freedom from many illnesses and diseases by early detection and cure—has, up to this time, been almost completely ignored by the West's medical establishment.

This analysis barely scratches the surface of pulse diagnosis and the possibilities it presents. The pulses may be checked not only at the wrists, but also at the neck, abdomen, feet, temples, back, and a number of places near the heart. These are less frequently used than the wrists in acupuncture but involve equally complex systems of pulse qualities and produce comparable results.

Three other methods of diagnosis supplement what an acupuncturist learns from the pulses. In childern the pulses are often too weak to yield meaningful answers about illness. And since very young childern cannot give reliable answers to questions, pediatrics is called the "mute specialization" in China. The doctor relies on only two of the four diagnostic methods to find out what is wrong with a child. The other two, sphygmology and questioning, are often useless. He bases his treatment on inspection and on hearing and smelling.

Inspection is the second most important method of diagnosis available to the acupuncturist. He learns far more from looking at a patient than a Western physician does. Since all the organs have counterparts on the body's surface, the acupuncturist who is well trained observes subtle changes in his patient's skin and body openings. Inspection is less exact than pulse diagnosis, but it often reveals the general area of the body a Chinese doctor should investigate fully.

The patient's tongue and eyes provide a multitude of information to the experienced Chinese doctor. The eyes are the orifice of the liver. Since the liver is the first organ in the order of correspondencies, the eyes are divided into many parts, each of which relates to a separate organ. The upper eyelid, for example, tells the condition of the spleen, and the white of the eye reveals the state of the lungs. The tongue is divided in a similar manner. Its root corresponds to the kidneys, and its two sides relate to the liver. The acupuncturist also studies a patient's coloring, since different colors correlate with various organs.

Hearing and *smelling* also tell the acupuncturist far more than they reveal to Western physicians. A Chinese doctor listens for subtle changes in a patient's voice that indicate illness, and attempts to find body odors that hint at the center of a Yin-Yang disturbance. Certain sounds that sick people often make correspond to different organs. Weeping relates to the lungs, laughter to the heart, groaning to the liver, singing to the stomach, and sobbing to the bladder.

Questioning allows the acupuncturist to discover facts about a patient that no other form of diagnosis will reveal. Since the four directions (five, counting the center) are related to the organs, people from different regions are more prone to some illnesses than to others. Acupuncture treatments that work for a patient from the South have little effect on a patient from the North. Questions about a patient's life help the acupuncturist learn how active he is, what kinds of weather he is exposed to, what foods he eats, and what type of daily schedule he follows. None of a Chinese doctor's questions are frivolous; they all relate to Yin and Yang, and so to the body's health.

When his diagnosis is complete, the acupuncturist immediately picks up his needles and begins the treatment. He does not take long deciding where the needles will be placed or how long they will be left in—because of another unique feature of traditional Chinese medicine. Once the doctor has found the center of a Yin-Yang imbalance and has determined its severity, the treatment has already been indicated. The pulse diagnosis has told him the exact nature of the imbalance. The system of meridians and points instructs him in the use of the needles, telling him at what points they must be inserted for every different illness and disease.

From the shelf in his shop reserved for his needles, the acupuncturist chooses the proper needles for the job they must perform. Today only stainless steel needles are used in Europe, the Soviet Union, and much of China. Before the advent of modern alloys, needles were made of gold, silver, copper, or brass, and before that of flint and other kinds of stone. European, Russian, and most Chinese acupuncturists use only three types of needles now, all the same except in length. Originally there were nine different types, each with a special use. They are:

1. The *Ch'an chen,* or chisel needle, 1.6 inches long. Its end is shaped like an arrowhead and has a sharply pointed tip. It is used in treating skin diseases.
2. The *Yuan chen,* or round needle, 1.6 inches long. It has an egg-shaped tip and cylindrical shaft. It is used for muscular massage and draining an excess of Ch'i.
3. The *Shih chen,* or spoon needle, 3.5 inches long. It has a rounded end, and is only used when the pulses are strong.

火長毫圓鈹鋒鍉圓鑱
針針針利針針針針針

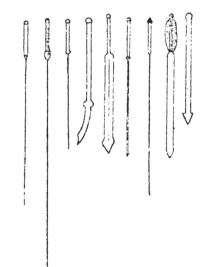

FIG. 44 THE NINE NEEDLES OF ACUPUNCTURE

4. The *Feng chen*, or lance needle, 1.6 inches long. It makes a large hole and is only used in chronic diseases that require drastic measures. Acupuncturists rarely need it.
5. The *Pi chen*, or stiletto needle, 4 inches long, 1.5 inches wide. It is shaped like the blade of a curved sword, and is also used in chronic diseases.
6. The *Yuan Li chen*, or round sharp needle, 1.6 inches long. It is used to relieve pain and paralysis.
7. The *Hao chen*, or soft hair needle, 3.6 inches long. It is used to stop pain and cure paralysis and numbness. It is often plunged into the body up to its full length.
8. The *Chang chen*, or long needle, 7 inches long. It is very sharp and used to relieve pain deep inside the body. It is also used in cancer treatments.
9. The *Ho chen*, or fire needle, 4 inches long. It is used to treat cases of poisoning and to relieve swelling (see Figure 44).

Only two or three of the ancient needles were used to prick the acupuncture points. Some were early surgical instruments, such as the *Pi chen* which doctors used to drain abscesses. Modern needles are from one to three inches long, very slender—almost as narrow as a human hair—and flexible. They are as effective as the old needles at the acupuncture points, but do not have as wide a variety of uses. When acupuncture was the only form of medical treatment in China, except for a few herb remedies dispensed by alchemists, all illnesses were treated with the old-style needles. Even now they are not obsolete in China. Thousands of acupuncturists trained before the Communists took power continue to treat patients with them. When a new generation of Chinese doctors completely replaces the old, the nine needles will likely become a part of history.

As China slowly modernizes, the shop of the local physician may well slip into the past too. But for many years to come, it will remain standing in thousands of villages, where it serves the needs of the people well. Even when the last shop is replaced by a gleaming clinic, Chinese doctors will continue to take the pulses, inspect, question, and listen to their patients, apply the correspondencies, and choose the proper needles. Before they can pierce the skin and return Yin and Yang to balance, they must consider one more set of factors: the laws of acupuncture.

CHAPTER IX

THE LAWS OF ACUPUNCTURE

Man is Heaven and Earth in Miniature.

—*Chinese Proverb*

FOUR RULES govern how the acupuncturist chooses to treat a patient. They are needed for two reasons. First, as Western medicine knows and too often ignores, any kind of medical treatment, whether by drugs or needles, will produce side effects. Drugs used to stimulate the heart often alter the body's function in other ways. The same thing happens in acupuncture. The needles may return one organ's Yin and Yang to balance but at the same time disturb the equilibrium in another. An acupuncturist must be aware of these possibilities and avoid them. Second, a diseased organ may be so far out of balance that the use of needles on it presents a danger of further damage. Acupuncture will intensify the illness rather than cure it. The laws provide a method of treating such .an organ by puncturing a meridian that belongs to a different organ.

The four laws of acupuncture are called the *Mother-Son* law, the *Husband-Wife* law, the *Noon-Midnight* law, and the *Law of the Five Elements.*

The *Mother-Son* law depends on the orderly flow of Ch'i through the meridians. Ch'i begins its cycle of the

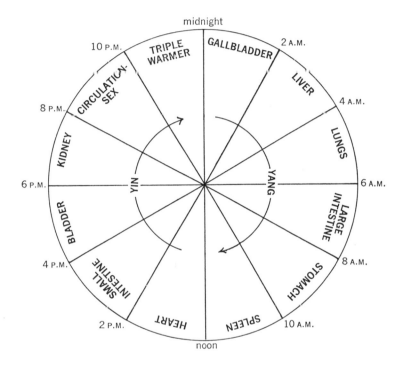

FIG. 45 NOON-MIDNIGHT LAW OF ACUPUNCTURE

In the practice of acupuncture, doctors choose certain times of day to treat the various organs. Yin organs respond best at the time of day they are most active, according to the organ-clock above. Yang organs follow the same principle. A corollary of the law states that treating one organ will also affect the organ opposite it on the clock.

body in the lungs. From there, in order, it flows through the large intestine, stomach, spleen, heart, small intestine, bladder, kidneys, circulation-sex, Triple Warmer, gallbladder, and liver meridians. According to the law, a meridian that precedes another is its "mother." One that directly follows it is its "son." The stomach meridian is the son of the large intestine and the mother of the spleen. The spleen is the mother of the heart, and so on. When an acupuncturist wishes to increase the activity of Yin or Yang in one organ, he can do it by stimulating the organ that is its mother. He can decrease Yin or Yang in the same way. The law has many corollaries that operate on the same principle.

The *Husband-Wife* law also deals with the relationship between the meridians, but in a different way. On each of the wrists, the pulses used in diagnosis are parallel to pulses on the other wrist. The small intestine pulse, for example, is felt in the superficial position at the *ts'un* section (see Figure 43) of the left wrist. On the right wrist, the pulse of the large intestine occupies the same position at the same spot. The left wrist is the Yang, or "husband" wrist; the right wrist is the Yin, or "wife" wrist. Needling a meridian that corresponds to an organ with a "husband" pulse will affect the parallel "wife" pulse. In a healthy body, the "husband" pulses dominate (are stronger than) the "wife" pulses. The acupuncturist must be careful not to upset this relationship when he applies the needles.

The *Noon-Midnight* law governs the effect of the time of day on the needles. Figure 45 is an organ-clock of the body showing when each of the twelve organs is most active. Organs are more responsive to treatment at the times of day they are most energetic, based on whether they are Yin or Yang. The stomach, a Yang organ, will respond to stimulation, an increase in Yang, best at about 8 a.m., a Yang time of day. If the stomach

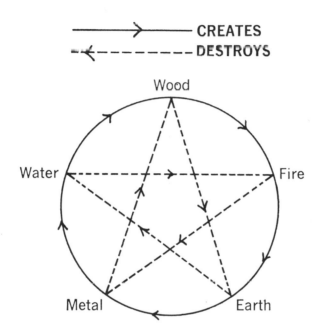

FIG. 46 THE FIVE ELEMENTS

The entire universe is constantly changing, according to Chinese philosophy, based on the interactions of the Five Elements, as the chart shows them. The creative and destructive processes also go on in man following the same cycle.

is stimulated, its opposite on the clock, the circulation-sex organ, will also be stimulated. But if the acupuncturist treats it at 10 p.m., the result will be slight, both because 10 p.m. is a Yin time of day and because the stomach is a Yang organ. Acupuncturists often schedule treatments to correspond with this law.

The *Law of the Five Elements* follows the interaction of the elements in nature (see Figure 46). If the Ch'i activity in the spleen is increased, for example, the organ it generates according to the theory of the elements, the lungs, will also show an increase in activity. But the organ the spleen destroys, the kidneys, will experience a decrease in Yin-Yang activity. The other organs follow the same rule. The interrelationships of the organs have a powerful effect on the body, and in his treatments no acupuncturist will ignore the law controlling those interrelationships.

None of the laws reveal how, specifically, the acupuncturist increases or decreases Yin or Yang with his needles. If he needs to increase the Yin in the large intestine, or decrease it, or change the activity of the Yang in the organ, how, using the same needles, can he differentiate between them? He does it by the way he inserts the needles and by using them either hot or cold. To stimulate Yang, the acupuncturist inserts the needle slowly, withdraws it rapidly, and massages the spot after the needle is taken out. He stimulates the Yin in the same way. To calm the Yang or Yin, he inserts the needle rapidly, withdraws it slowly, and does not massage the spot afterward. Yin and Yang are distinguished by hot and cold; cold needles are used for Yin treatments, hot ones for Yang. If, as he inserts the needle, the acupuncturists twists it clockwise, Yang will be influenced. A counterclockwise motion will produce a change in Yin.

The patient's pulses determine the length of time the needle is left in the meridian. While the needles are in the acupuncture points, the doctor feels the pulses that have shown abnormal characteristics. As soon as the irregularities disappear, the needle is withdrawn.

The number of needles an acupuncturist uses depends on the illness and on his skill. Some serious diseases require up to forty-two needles, all inserted at a single session. Other illnesses can be cured with one needle. An expert acupuncturist needs only one needle to cure a toothache, while a mediocre practitioner may use eight or nine.

Common illnesses can usually be cured in one session with the acupuncturist. Chinese doctors believe that if a medication is good enough to cure an ailment, it need only be used once. Western medicine, because it is a much less exact science then acupuncture, often involves massive, repeated doses of drugs to treat an illness. Acupunturists feel, quite logically, that they can discover the cause of any ailment through pulse diagnosis, treat it immediately with needles, and see the results of their treatment at once. The treatment need not end until the illness is cured. Severe disturbances in Yin and Yang that are difficult to cure may take more than one application of the needles and so may complex diseases. Some of the newer uses of acupuncture, such as the treatment of nerve deafness in children, call for up to forty applications of the needles, but those instances are rare. Expert acupuncturists use their needles only once in a great majority of the illnesses they treat.

Acupuncturists will not treat ailments that they know do not respond to the needles. Most communicable diseases caused by bacteria are immune to needling, but this in no way lessens the importance of acupuncture as a form of treatment. In ancient China, many of the communicable diseases familiar to the West were unknown. Syphilis was brought to China by Western colonists in 1504.* Strong evidence exists that both the plague and smallpox came to China from India and the Middle East. Acupuncture was invented before China knew of these and many other diseases. For three thousand years Chinese people believed that the world ended at their borders, as did Europeans. Acupuncture had no provision for illnesses that might come from other countries, since no other countries were known. Modern hindsight sees this as a flaw in the medical system. To the Chinese, it was merely being practical. Some illnesses defy any cure. Acupuncture alleviates the symptoms of these as easily as Western medicine, and in many cases with better results.

The Chinese physician, as he treats his patients, gives a very different impression from his Western counterpart. He approaches each illness, minor or major, with utter confidence. No doubt about the efficiency of his treatment crosses his mind: his manner is not a facade erected to keep his patients happy and give them hope. Instead, it reflects as true belief that there is no disease, no affliction known to mankind, that the physician, properly applying acupuncture and other healing techniques, will be unable to cure.

The entire universe, he feels, works in such a precise, orderly fashion, that it contains no mysteries beyond his scope of understanding. This is not arrogance, but a rich feeling of association between man and nature. Because no supreme power, no Lord of Hosts, created the world, the forces behind life and death and illness and health are not beyond man's comprehension. They are, in the form of Ch'i, present in every living creature, every tree and flower, every puff of wind and drop of rain.

The acupuncturist sees the lives of his patients as

* The carriers were Dutch explorers, as many Western historians have recorded in histories of China and the Netherlands.

integral parts of the universe. He brings his patients back to health not only for their own sake and happiness, but so that the whole world may function properly. Every needle the acupuncturist twirls between his fingers bears the heavy weight of universal harmony in its slim, pointed end.

CHAPTER X

HERB MEDICINE AND OTHER HEALING ARTS

A happy mind is medicine; no better prescription exists.

—Chinese proverb

AN ELEPHANT'S skin, burned to ashes, helps open wounds heal. Powdered turtle shells strengthen weak kidneys and dissolve gallstones. Swallow's nest soup revives the sick and elderly. Pig's kidneys stop pain and ease inflammations. Pulverized rhinoceros' horn draws the poison from snakebites. Quicksilver destroys intestinal worms. Frogs' skins cure dropsy. Seahorses reduce goiters. Dragonflies increase sexual potency.

Your family physician is not likely to prescribe any of these remedies, nor will you find them on the shelves at your corner drugstore—unless you happen to be in China. There thousands of physicians rely on many of them in daily practice, and they can be bought over the counter in every village pharmacy.

These remedies—and hundreds more like them—are part of China's legacy of folk medicine, the richest in the world. As preposterous as some of them sound, they are potent, effective, and popular. And not as far-fetched as their ingredients suggest.

Frogs' skins, for example, not only cure dropsy, but also provide a secretion used to treat dog bites. Frogs'

166

blood is mixed with sugar and eaten as a way of removing metal objects accidentally swallowed. Chinese doctors have used both the skins and blood successfully for thousands of years. Recently Western chemists isolated a substance in frogs' skins that is almost identical to digitalis. Western physicians treat certain heart conditions with digitalis, and frogs' skins may very well be an effective cure for dropsy. The main source of digitalis in the West is the foxglove plant. Chinese doctors happen to use the root of the foxglove in herb remedies given to some heart patients. Large doses of digitalis save many lives in both China and the West. It is one of the safest, most effective heart stimulants ever discovered.

Is the parallel a coincidence? Hardly. Chinese doctors began developing drugs three thousand years before Western physicians did. They lacked the scientific methods of research and the laboratory equipment that have enabled Western physicians to develop drugs rapidly and efficiently in the last century. But they were no less dedicated or conscientious in their work than Western doctors. Ultimately, as every nation's medical men must, they built a body of drug prescriptions based on success in treating illness with them.

Chinese remedies came from nature, from the plants and animals early physicians found readily available. They had no means of extracting medicinal substances from roots or leaves or skins. The ingredients in their prescriptions have never been as refined or pure as those used in the West. Often, however, as with digitalis, they contain the same basic drugs. Yet any similarity between Western prescriptions and traditional Chinese herb remedies ends there.

Herbalists use many more ingredients in each prescription than Western doctors do. They prescribe drugs on a completely different basis, using formulas and rules of medication as alien to Western medicine as acupuncture. Their art centers on the Chinese theory of the universe, and on the belief that imbalances in Yin and Yang cause man's physical ills.

As with acupuncture treatments, Chinese drug remedies are suited to each patient and the illness he has. Doctors who practice both acupuncture and herb medicine use pulse diagnosis in deciding what ingredients will return Yin and Yang to balance. Those who specialize in herb medicine alone either study the pulse or perform calculations of other kinds that are equally intricate and precise. Unlike Western drugs, which usually come pre-mixed and ready to dispense, most herb remedies must be compounded for each patient a doctor treats. Some prescriptions contain thirty or more different ingredients; others combine only two or three. Over the centuries a few prescriptions have become standard in certain illnesses, much as aspirin is a universal Western curative for pain. Chinese doctors and medicine shops made up batches of these remedies, usually in pill form, and dispensed or sold them to local peasants. Those offered by "doctors" of uncertain qualifications, or in open-air markets by vendors working from portable stands, were and are of doubtful effectiveness. As long as there has been illness in the world, quacks as well as professional physicians have flourished. In China, they were the first entrepreneurs of patent medicines.

One of the pills long favored by the Chinese people is called the "Nine Fairies" remedy. It is supposed to have life-saving qualities, but has been more normally used to treat infected sores and boils. Some of its ingredients are cinnabar, flowers of sulphur, olibanum, myrrh, camphor, dragon's blood, copper sulphate, musk, alum, yellow lead, centipedes, earthworms, silkworms, plum flowers, white jade dust, and snails. The Chinese people take it very seriously; many of them will swear by its effectiveness, even today. Hundreds of other, equally unusual remedies line the shelves of village medicine shops and the cases of street-corner hawkers. Some are used by reputable physicians, minus ingredients such as dragon's blood and centipedes. The bulk of them belong in the category of old wives' tales about hanging garlic around the neck to ward off disease (a popular Eastern European custom). Yet the patent medicine herb remedies cannot be dismissed so easily. They are the cause of most Western misconceptions about Chinese folk medicine.

China's masses have been superstitious since the dawn of recorded history, and naturally so. Viewing the universe as an integral entity of man, nature, and lifeless objects—a highly organized sphere filled with millions of interlocking parts—the people were bound to look for omens of good or bad fortune in their natural surroundings. They believed fervently that nature dictated the course of their lives in everything from farming to health to social situations. A majority of the people has always been illiterate, even counting the millions who have received an elementary education under Mao Tse-tung's government. Lacking the skills needed to comprehend Tao, the way to mastering one's destiny and health, the peasant masses became superstitious about the forces of nature. They created talismans against the evils brought by changes in nature's rhythms. Many can be seen today in the Chinese sections of large Western cities. They are the charms and wall plaques and wind chimes and lanterns that make up a kind of superstition-for-profit capitalism (some have been created strictly for the tourist trade and are far more authentic).

In China, the talismans took many forms, varying from place to place. Red or yellow pieces of paper bearing written warnings against evil influences were popular for centuries. They were burned at altars or hung on doors and walls. Firecrackers were used the same way, and jade was considered a near-perfect means of keeping fortune shining on its owner. In medicine, the superstitions allowed a class of faith-healers to evolve, who were in no way related to professional physicians. Commonly, the healers would write on a piece of paper held over a bowl of water while chanting for the sickness to leave. The ailing peasant then drank the water, believing that his illness would soon abate. When it did not, he blamed himself, not the healer, for being unable to restore the harmony that ruled health.

Close upon these healers came the patent medicines, and in much the same vein. Doctors have always been scarce in China, especially before this century's political upheavals. The time of a true physician was valuable, and no matter how devoted he was to healing the sick, the number of people he could treat was limited. The years of study, coupled with the difficulty of leaving the land for any academic pursuit, kept the number of trained medical professionals low. Healers gleaned what they could from the real practice of medicine and set up shop with their questionable pills and potions and useless charms and incantations. Superstition and lack of any other recourse drew the people to them.

Every nation has had its faith-healers, mystics, and quasi-doctors. In a broad sense, the corporate giants of today that manufacture non-prescription remedies, such as the popular cold capsules, are their modern descendants. As science developed and the people attained a high degree of education and knowledge, the nations outgrew early superstitions and healers. China did not enter a scientific age until the middle of this century. The old beliefs prevailed for thousands of years and became ingrained in the cultural heritage passed from generation to generation. Education never became the right of the masses; it still is not, even under an enlightened government. Survival, mastering the land so that enough food was produced to feed the people, commanded a much higher priority. The professions suffered most, especially medicine, since the common people believed deeply in the power of remedies available from their local healers. Drugs of doubtful worth continued to be the largest source of the average peasant's medical care. Faith-healers and patent medicine dealers thrived. They became respectable "doctors" for millions of people.

Early Western observers garnered their opinions of Chinese drugs and doctors from these healers. Understandably, and regrettably, the honored and respected art of the true Chinese physicians went unnoticed. It seemed to be only a more complex, but equally useless, form of faith-healing. The Yellow Man was baffling enough, in his preoccupations with social customs and civility, and his riches were waiting to be tapped. Why bother delving into his form of medicine, which was obviously just superstition and nonsense? Travelers to the Orient brought home tales of healers who drew Chinese characters in the air above a dying patient, then pronounced him cured. Merchants and explorers and missionaries dismissed what they saw of Chinese medicine as the primitive rites of a backward race. But what they viewed was only one side of a two-headed coin—the dark side.

Chiselled on the other face was the image of the erudite, brilliant masters of Chinese medicine, dedicated physicians who learned and extended the knowledge accumulated over thousands of years. These men— and they all were men—agreed with the Western visitors about China's faith-healers. They saw the "Nine Fairies" pill in the same light, but they also knew that acupuncture and herb remedies were effective forms of medical treatment. Herbalists relied on the ancient systems that made their practice possible because they had no more scientific method of treating illness. Little could be done for the people who insisted on visiting street-corner healers and patent medicine stands. Only more doctors would help, and the poverty that dominated Chinese life made that impossible. More lucrative professions beckoned the rich men's sons who might become doctors, and few of them possessed the intelligence needed to pass the government examinations. The quacks that operated on the fringe of the medical profession stole the herbalists' remedies and added to them to satisfy the people's superstition. At least in that way some reliable drugs reached the masses. Often, exactly that happened, and most Chinese patent medicines that contain such things as dragon's blood and centipedes have one or two ingredients that really do help cure illness. Herb remedies came to have a dual identity, one associated with the strange uses made of them by faith-healers and quacks, the other linked to their real worth when prescribed by a true physician.

From their first encounters with it, Western medical experts refused to believe that Chinese medicine had any worth. Acupuncture with its mysterious principles and unsanitary conditions ran against the teachings of European, Russian, and American medical schools. The Chinese accepted the label "unscientific" because it was true. The West equated it with the word "inferior." The effectiveness of traditional Chinese medicine could not be taken at face value by Western doctors; nothing can unless it proves sound according to approved scientific measurements. So what if hundreds of millions of people were being treated and cured by acupuncture and herb remedies? Traditional medicine had no basis in the Western medical establishment's system of values. It was written off as something midway between voodoo and sorcery.

China's most popular folk medicine, *ginseng,* is an excellent example of a traditional herb remedy's dual identity. Ginseng comes from a plant shaped like a human figure. Its Chinese name is *jen shen,* or *man root.* Early Chinese doctors believed, as did doctors in Europe, that a plant's shape would influence its curative powers. A plant shaped like a human heart would strengthen the heart. One shaped like the kidneys would relieve kidney diseases. The ginseng root should, therefore, be effective in treating many illnesses.

Other nations carried the principle, called the *Doctrine of Signatures,* even further. European folklore contains the legend that eating the liver of tigers, where courage supposedly dwells, makes a man brave. In the Middle Ages warriors often gathered the night before a battle to cut up freshly slaughtered animals and eat the raw livers, as well as drink their blood. The practice was also common in China for a few centuries.

Chinese people have used ginseng to cure anemia, depression, asthma, colds, eye trouble, exhaustion, heart attacks, headaches, indigestion, impotence, nausea, rheumatism, frigidity, listlessness, dizziness, and emotional upsets, among other illnesses. The list of ailments thought responsive to the wonder root is practically endless. And the Chinese are not alone in their respect for the man root. Ginseng sells briskly in European and American health food stores. It is added to cosmetics in the West, and thousands of Westerners drink ginseng tea or tonic every morning to pep up their days and cure any illnesses lurking in the background. Korean-grown ginseng can be bought in Europe and the United States in capsule form, mixed with honey, and as a liqueur. Pure ginseng extract sells for two hundred dollars a pound, making it one of the two or three most expensive plants in the world.

Western devotees of the man root believe that it eases tension, soothes upset stomachs, makes the skin silky and glowing, and attracts the opposite sex. Ginseng liqueur, claim some people, gives a greater high than the purest marijuana. A few Chinese believers wear the root around their necks as a dual charm: it wards off illness and increases sexual attraction.

In China every village medicine shop carries ginseng, and millions buy it daily for any—or all—of its supposed powers. China's physicians use it too, but in a very different way. They prescribe ginseng, in varying concentrations, as a mild sedative, tension reliever, or pain depressant. Mixed with an extract from the root of a type of loco weed, it is taken before meals to prevent upset stomachs. Combined with honey and cinnamon, it stimulates blood circulation. A broth made of ginseng and bamboo leaves works as a mild sedative. Herbalists add it to the complicated prescriptions given to very sick patients for those qualities, but they make no claim that it is a miracle drug capable of curing dozens of illnesses.

Because ginseng is so popular, chemists in the West have analyzed its components. It includes a resin, starch, tannin, bitters, and saponin, among other ingredients. Saponin is part of a group of chemicals called glyoxides, which Western doctors often use to treat high blood pressure. The relationship of high blood pressure to tension, insomnia, stomach problems, and hyperactivity is well known to doctors in every country. Chinese herbalists closely approximate the Western use of ginseng's most potent ingredient when they mix their remedies. Fact, whether in the practice of Chinese or Western medicine, overcomes the fantasy of faddists or faith-healers.

Chinese doctors rarely use ginseng alone. They compound prescriptions containing it according to the needs of each patient and the ancient rules of herb medicine. The rules are part of a system dating back to at least the second century A.D. and the celebrated doctor Chang Chung-ching, the Hippocrates of the East.

One of Dr. Chang's major works was the *Illnesses Caused by Cold*. It listed over one hundred herb remedies mixed by a method called the *Doctrine of the Seven Recipes.* Chang did not create the doctrine; he attributed it to Emperor Shen Nung, the legendary ruler who had a transparent stomach and authored the *Pen Ts'ao.* Chang expended the system to provide extensive rules for mixing herb remedies. He viewed herbs and animal substances the same way Chinese doctors saw the body, as a mirror of society. Chang divided medicinal herbs into four categories; emperor, minister, chancellor, and ambassador. This closely resembles Western principles for combining drugs, where there is a basic curative that rules the prescription (emperor), an aid to the basic drug, or adjuvant (minister), a corrective ingredient that sets the healing process in motion (chancellor), and a vehicle for the prescription (ambassador).

Most Chinese herb remedies contain all these ingredients in varying proportions. The *Doctrine of the Seven Recipes* helps doctors decide what the proportion of each should be, based on how severe the Yin-Yang disturbance is. The seven recipes are:

1. *Ch'i fang,* or odd-numbered recipe. These prescriptions contain an odd number of ingredients, such as two emperor herbs and three minister herbs. In nearly all prescriptions one chancellor and one ambassador is added. *Ch'i fang* prescriptions increase the activity of Yang. They are used only in Yin illnesses, where Yang needs strengthening. They are never prescribed when Yin symptoms are present.

2. *Go fang,* or even-numbered recipe. An even number of emperor and minister drugs are used. *Go fang* prescriptions are Yin remedies, used when Yang is too active.

3. *Ta fang*, or great recipe. When an illness is serious, with many symptoms, an herbalist will prescribe a *Ta fang* remedy. There are few of

them, and they are very powerful, sometimes
containing small amounts of poisonous herbs.

4. *Hsao fang*, or little recipe. Simple illnesses,
with the patient displaying only one symptom,
require *Hsao fang*. Only two or three ingredients are compounded to make them.

5. *Huan fang*, or slow recipe. These are gentle
remedies, used when a patient's condition is too
poor to stand strong drugs. They contain herbs
that build strength.

6. *Chi fang*, or emergency recipe. The effects of
Chi fang prescriptions are immediate. Patients
near death are given them to increase the activity of Ch'i in the body.

7. *Ch'ung fang*, or repeated recipe. Complicated
illnesses sometimes require prescriptions that
will work on a number of organs at the same
time. These remedies contain many herbs and
are taken several times.

The *Doctrine of the Seven Recipes* simplifies a physician's work, but only after he has located the exact spot
at which a Yin-Yang imbalance has occurred. The
principles of Chinese anatomy and physiology are the
same in acupuncture and herb medicine, as are the
diagnostic techniques. Many Chinese physicians practice both because the basic training for them—medical
school, in Western terms—is the same.

Acupuncture alone requires only one herb, the leaves
of *Artemesia vulgaris,* the Chinese mugwort, or wormwood, tree. When an illness calls for a "hot" (Yang)
treatment, small piles of *ai yen,* as it is called in
Chinese, or *moxa*, as it is known in English, are burned
on the skin after the needle is withdrawn. Some acupuncturists place the piles of moxa on the end of the
needle while it is in place, thus heating the acupuncture
point. Moxabustion may be used alone to treat a few
illnesses. It is considered extremely effective in relieving

pain when a woman is giving birth, and in treating eye diseases. Used improperly, it can be dangerous; some acupuncture points are never treated with moxa, nor is moxa used on patients with severe Yang illnesses.

The aromas filling the air in the shops of village physicians come from the herbs they use to compound prescriptions. Some are found in plants common throughout the world. Others are peculiar to China. They are seldom prescribed, or useful, alone. A trained physician's expertise is needed to mix them according to the *Doctrine of the Seven Recipes*. The following list includes only a few of them—herbalists use nearly a thousand—and the illnesses they are helpful in treating:

An hsih liu: pomegranate. The bark of the pomegranate tree kills tapeworms and stops diarrhoea.

T'ao: peach. Stones of peaches relieve rheumatism and constipation.

Jou to k'ou: nutmeg. Useful as a heart stimulant.

San ken: Russian mulberry. Reduces swellings and ulcers.

Lien tze: lotus flower. Reduces fevers and heals skin diseases.

Lian ch'ao: weeping forsythia. Reduces swellings and kills intestinal worms.

T'ien hsih li: Chinese chestnut. Effective in treating rheumatism.

T'ien men tung: asparagus. Relieves coughs and aches in the arms and legs.

Chu hsin: bamboo. Has many uses, including as a stomach-soothing broth.

P'ai t'ou kou: cardamom. A member of the ginger family; reduces fever and restores strength.

Kuei: cinnamon. Relieves flatulence.

Ch'ing hao: tarragon. Reduces fever.

Ch'uan liu: purple willow. Part of a rheumatism remedy.

P'u kung yin: dandelion. Has many applications,

including treatment of venereal diseases and ulcers.
Ju hsiang: pistachio. Used externally in plasters.
Hu t'ao: Persian walnut. Used to treat kidney ailments.
Kan ts'ao: licorice. Pain reliever, fever reducer, and ingredient in most prescriptions.
Ma huang: Chinese ephedra. Effective in heart diseases, headaches, eye inflammations, and bronchitis.
Mu fang chi: snailseed. Relieves asthma.
Hsi hsin: wild ginger. Cures hearing defects.
Fan hsieh yeh: an effective laxative; no English equivalent.
Sheng ma: skunk bugbane. Calms nerves and eases headaches.
Nu p'ang tze: great burdock. Cures skin rashes.
Tu chung: Chinese rubber tree. Leaves ground to make a powder effective against hemorrhoids.
Huang ch'ang shan: effective in cases of recurrent malaria; no English equivalent.

Acupunture and herb medicine form the nucleus of traditional Chinese medicine, but they are not its only forms. Many traditional physicians use Chinese massage to treat specific illnesses. Some forms of it may be classified as medicine; others approximate Western massage techniques that concentrate on relaxing and toning the body. A few Chinese physicians, and many Japanese physicians, claim to produce the same results by pressing acupuncture points as by piercing them with needles. Their claims have never been verified, except when spot-pressing, as it is called, is used to relieve minor pains by interfering with nerve functions through finger pressure on the skin. Relief is quick in such cases, but temporary. The cause of the pain is not at all affected.

Another massage technique involves working the skin and muscles with the thumb and first three fingers, while the heel of the hand remains stationary. Zones of the body are gently manipulated, depending on the type of illness. The *Nei Ching* mentions this type of massage and gives specific uses for it. During the T'ang dynasty (618-907 A.D.), it became extremely popular. Institutes were established throughout China to teach it, but not as a replacement for herb medicine or acupuncture. Knowing the relationship between tension and illness, many Chinese doctors prescribe some form of massage for all their patients.

Chinese physicians often prescribe another means of body conditioning for their patients: physical culture. There are several different Chinese exercise systems, some more complicated than acupuncture. All are based on the Chinese belief in Ch'i as the motivating force of life and in the necessity to control Ch'i through proper care of the body. Ch'i is sometimes erroneously translated as breath because of the method of attaining superior health by controlling one's breathing. Much like the Indian Yoga, Chinese exercises try to bring about a tranquil state of mind that will allow the body to function properly. Unlike Yoga, the exercises require achievement of no particular physical agility. They do not exhaust the body, or even place any undue strain on it. Instead, they keep the flow of Ch'i constant and strong, thereby insuring good health.

The earliest Chinese exercise form was the game of the Five Animals, invented by Hua T'o in the second century A.D. Man imitated a bear, a stag, a monkey, a tiger, and a crane in order to make his body supple and natural. Perfection of the exercises insured a long life, hopefully one hundred years, which Hua T'o thought was the natural limit.

The Five Animals game was divided into two parts, as are most Chinese gymnastics. First came the *ch'i chung,* in which the body was kept immobile and proper breathing was practiced. The player concentrated on ridding himself of poor breathing habits. Respiration should be silent, easy, and slow, placing no undue strain on the vital organs. A raspy, noisy, or labored breathing means that the person's mind is not at ease. It may be filled with contradicting thoughts that can lead to illness.

After *ch'i chung* came *t'ai chi chua,* the mobile part of the game. The five animals were imitated in series while the exerciser breathed properly. The body would become limber and the mind tranquil.

The name *t'ai chi chua* comes from the symbol for Yin and Yang, a circle bisected by an "S" and called the *t'ai chi tu.* Later gymnasts developed a series of exercises based on rotating the arms and legs in circles while the trunk of the body remained still. By duplicating the Yin-Yang symbol the body was brought into harmony with the universe. Medically, Chinese exercises are on a par with massage. They relax the body, leading to good health.

Traditional Chinese physicians use massage and physical culture in the daily practice of medicine, but they rely on acupuncture and herb medicine to treat illness and disease. Their effectiveness is difficult to doubt; they have survived millennia of trials and have retained the respect and faith of China's masses. At any stage in history Chinese culture has been significantly more developed than the West's, except in science. China's value systems and customs have always differed with the Western world's, and always will because of the different natural philosophy each has. Most Western people, for example, wear black to funerals, the color of death and mystery and despair. Chinese people wear white, because death is not necessarily a tragic event. The human spirit enters the line of revered ancestors when the body dies. It continues to live in the bodies of descendants. Death is not mysterious. Despair has no place.

This is but a tiny shred from the fabric of China's

culture, and the differences of that culture from the West's. But the Chinese people know that as the world grows smaller, they must keep pace with the West, especially in science. China has entered the nuclear age. With the aid of other communist nations, she has created and exploded an atomic bomb. Her people have assimilated much of the technology brought by the modern age. Hidden behind the Great Wall, the mountains, and the sea, China moves swiftly into the present. The turmoil between old and new, between China's unique view of the universe and the West's, rages constantly. The Dragon must stop breathing fire. It will be replaced by a nuclear-powered electric generator as a source of light and heat.

Chinese medicine has fallen in step with the long march toward today. Western medical techniques are becoming commonplace. Inoculations against contagious diseases are carried out on a huge scale. Hundreds of millions of people feel the prick of a different kind of needle, one on the end of a syringe. For most, it is their first brush with Western medicine. They accept it, less out of faith or trust in it than because Chairman Mao has proclaimed it necessary.

As the techniques of Western medicine become more and more available to the average Chinese citizen, acupuncture must face the ultimate test. Will it survive the onslaught of the best medical treatment and knowledge the West has to offer? So far, the answer is yes.

APPENDIX I

A GUIDE TO CHINESE PRONUNCIATION

The Chinese language contains many sounds that are extremely difficult—if not impossible—to render into English. Western Sinologists have, however, constructed systems of Romanization that allow the reader to approximate the correct pronunciation of Chinese words. The most accurate of these is the Wade-Giles Romanization, which this book follows with one or two exceptions.

Following the rules below, any Chinese term or name in this work may be satisfactorily pronounced. Only those words or names which through wide popular use, have taken on English spellings outside the system do not follow the rules.

VOWELS:

a as in f*a*ther;
i as in mach*i*ne;
e as in t*e*n;
o as in *o*rder;
u as the double "o" in m*oo*n.

VOWEL COMBINATIONS:

ai as in *ai*sle;
ao as the *ow* in h*ow;*
ei as in *ei*ght;
ou as in sh*ou*lder;
ua as the *wa* in *wa*ter.

CONSONANTS:

k as the *g* in *g*o;
k' as the *c* in *c*at;
t as the *d* in *d*og;
t' as the *t* in *t*ime;
p as the *b* in *b*oy;
p' as the *p* in *p*ie;

185

ts and *tz* as the *ds* in bea*ds*;

ts 'and *tz*' as the *ts* in mee*ts*;

hs as *sh* in *sh*oe;

j as the *r* in *r*un—there is no true English equivalent for the sound in Chinese, and it is best pronounced as a simple *r* sound.

OTHER SOUNDS:

en as the *un* in b*un*;

u before *n* as a German umlaut—similar to the *u* in b*u*rn;

eng as the *ung* in r*ung*;

u before *ng* as a German umlaut;

uei as *w*ay;

uai as the *wi* in *wi*de;

ih as the *ir* in b*ir*d—again, no true English equivalent exists, and only an approximation can be made.

APPENDIX II

ILLNESSES AND DISEASES
TREATED BY ACUPUNCTURE

The following list of symptoms, illnesses, and diseases and the points acupuncturists pierce to alleviate them is drawn from both Chinese and Western sources. It is not in any way a complete listing, which would consume hundreds of pages and differ from authority to authority. Nor is it meant as a guide for amateurs. It is intended as an indication of the thousands of ailments acupuncturists treat, and where they insert their needles.

The appendix follows illustrations numbered 16 through 27, meridian by meridian. The numbers beneath those headings below refer to the corresponding points numbered in the illustrations.

Often a symptom or illness will be listed beside more than one acupuncture point. This is because many ailments require acupuncture at more than one point.

CIRCULATION-SEX
(Figure 16: Arm Absolute Yin Meridian)

1. Paralysis in arms and legs; blurred vision; fever accompanied by headache; pain in breasts; insufficient production of milk in mothers.
2. Bronchitis; blurred vision; coughing; heart pain; vomiting; anorexia.
3. Sterility; chorea; measles; cholera; hemiplegia; diarrhoea; excessive thirst; abdominal pains.
4. Nausea; hemorrhoids; failing memory; undue fear of people; lassitude; myocarditis; epistaxis.
5. Malaria; gastritis; vomiting; cholera; cramps in joints; excess vaginal discharge; irregular menstruation; insanity; neurasthenia.
6. Jaundice; irregular menstruation; enteritis; insomnia;

189

diarrhoea; epilepsy; heart palpitations; dizziness; headaches.
7. Weariness; insanity; depression; breast ulcers; dry fever; shortness of breath; intestinal ulcers; continuous laughter.
8. Blood in urine; hemorrhoids; indigestion; stomach pains; jaundice; writer's cramp; anger; depression.
9. High blood pressure; most Yang diseases; delirium; fainting spells; unconsciousness.

LIVER
(*Figure 17: Leg Absolute Yin Meridian*)
1. Gonorrhea; lumbago; headaches; stomach pains; sleepiness.
2. Hysteria; insanity; convulsions; madness; pain in loins; dry throat; insomnia; short temper; breast abscesses; dizziness; swollen joints; dry coughs.
3. Nausea; muscle spasms; pain in loins and abdomen; pale skin; constipation; vomiting.
4. Impotence; vaginal pain; urethritis; swollen abdomen.
5. Belching; irregular menstruation; inability to urinate; general feeling of coldness.
6. Numbness on skin; general weakness; pharyngitis; diarrhoea.
7. Rheumatism; painful joints; stiff joints.
8. Madness; paralysis in both legs; vaginal pain; irregular menstruation; fibroids; muscle cramps; madness.
9. Boils; back pains; irregular menstruation.
10. Inability to urinate; swollen abdomen.
11. Inability to conceive children.
12. Pain in penis and loins.
13. Jaundice; high blood pressure; flatulence; swollen abdomen; oedema; excessive weight loss.
14. Peritonitis; excessive thirst; difficulty in giving birth; coughing; general achiness in body.

TRIPLE WARMER
(*Figure 18: Arm Lesser Yang Meridian*)
1. Malaria; headache; poor vision; cholera; pyrexia.
2. Toothache; inability to concentrate; gingivitis; deafness; coldness in limbs.
3. Vertigo; dizziness; headaches; loss of coordination in fingers; dry fever; back pain.
4. Diabetes; muscular spasms; melancholy; shivering.

5. Infantile paralysis; high blood pressure; chest pains; undue fear; fever; toothache; influenza; colds.
6. Eczema; vomiting; pleurisy; pneumonia; cholera; swollen limbs; lockjaw; heart pains.
7. Epilepsy; slight deafness; nervous agitation.
8. Deafness; toothaches; lethargy; sleepiness.
9. Deafness; pharyngitis; toothache.
10. Insanity; bronchitis; lack of appetite; tinnitus; tonsillitis; headaches behind ear on one side.
11. Sides of body painful; yellow eyes; arms painful and stiff.
12. Vertigo; stiff neck; swollen arms.
13. Goiters; back and shoulder pains; stiff and painful arms.
14. Stiffness in arms and shoulders.
15. Inability to perspire; chest pain; stiff neck.
16. Pain in arms; sudden deafness; stiff neck; pain in arms and shoulders.
17. Mumps; toothache; facial paralysis; swollen lower jaw; muscle spasms in face and throat.
18. Convulsions; epilepsy; undue fear; vomiting; diarrhoea; blurred vision.
19. Convulsions; childhood fits; slight deafness.
20. Swollen gums; various diseases of the mouth, ears, and eyes.
21. Gingivitis; deafness; toothache; various diseases of the mouth.
22. Paralysis and spasms in face; swollen neck and jaws.
23. Madness; various diseases of the eyes; headaches.

GALLBLADDER
(*Figure 19: Leg Lesser Yang Meridian*)
1. Myopia; conjunctivitis; eyes tired and painful; color-blindness; headache.
2. Toothache; gingivitis; otorrhoea; deafness; convulsions.
3. Glaucoma; aversion to bright lights; vertigo; deafness.
4. Rheumatism; epilepsy; vertigo; deafness; toothache; poor and blurred vision.
5. Inability to perspire; eyes red and painful; face flushed; melancholy; toothache; epistaxis.
6. Facial swelling; dry fever; anorexia; headaches on one side of the head.
7. Various eye diseases; headaches; stiff neck.

8. Drunkenness; vomiting; severe headaches; depression; melancholy.
9. Insanity; epilepsy; toothache; headaches.
10. Deafness; toothache; coughing; numbness in neck and throat.
11. Dizziness; numbness in throat and mouth; various mouth diseases.
12. Insomnia; stiff neck; gingivitis; dark urine; insanity; epilepsy; paralysis in face; neck pain.
13. Undue fear; madness; epilepsy; vertigo; unconsciousness.
14. Nausea; headaches; various eye diseases.
15. Cerebral hemorrhage; pain in eyes; constant tearing of eyes; headache.
16. Vertigo; poor eyesight; various eye diseases; color-blindness.
17. Poor eyesight; vomiting; dizziness; toothache; gingivitis.
18. Inability to breathe through nose; headaches; general feeling of cold.
19. Weakness in body; severe headaches; dizziness.
20. Rheumatism; deafness; epistaxis; eye diseases; poisoning; poor vision; migraine headaches; dizziness; nasal disorders.
21. Ulcers; inability to speak; premature labor in pregnancy; head congestion; painful limbs; rheumatism.
22. Goiters; pleurisy; fullness in chest; general body weakness.
23. Depression; asthma; various respiratory diseases.
24. Muscle spasms; hiccoughs; slurred speech; vomiting; pain in swallowing.
25. Asthma; dark urine; diarrhoea; back pain; lumbago.
26. Heavy feeling in body; irregular menstruation; weak muscles.
27. Constipation; lower back pain.
28. Nephritis; intestinal diseases; oedema; lumbago; pain in legs.
29. Nephritis; cystitis; irregular menstruation; paralysis in arms.
30. Influenza; epilepsy; exhaustion; sciatica; rheumatism.
31. Sciatica; paralysis in children; muscular weakness in legs.
32. Muscle spasms; lack of coordination; lumbago; sciatica.
33. Legs swollen; stiffness in knee points; numbness.

34. Insanity; neurasthenia; lumbago; constipation; pharyngitis; poor circulation in legs.
35. Pleurisy; sciatica; coldness in feet and hands.
36. Insanity; paralysis; muscle spasms in legs; beriberi.
37. Diseases of the eyes; paralysis in legs; sudden madness.
38. Skin white and pasty; heart spasms; goiters; muscle spasms; pains in chest and legs; sciatica; coldness in lower part of body.
39. Acute appendicitis; lack of appetite; lack of coordination; rheumatism; diarrhoea; madness; bad temper; hemorrhoids.
40. Paralysis; general body weakness; muscle spasms; pain in legs; swollen neck; pain in lower body; difficulty in breathing.
41. Vertigo; fever; rheumatism; swelling in lower legs; conjunctivitis.
42. Breast ulcers; eye diseases.
43. Dry fever; vertigo; swollen limbs; head congestion; spasms in fingers and feet; pleurisy.
44. Insomnia; deafness; coughing; pain in eyes; nightmares; headache.

LUNGS
(*Figure 20: Arm Greater Yin Meridian*)

1. Pleurisy; stuttering; tonsillitis; insomnia; acne; bronchitis; night sweats; pneumonia.
2. Coughing tonsillitis; acne; heart disease; chest pains; shortness of breath.
3. Depression; vertigo; bronchitis; mental confusion; thirst; vomiting.
4. Chest pains; heart pains; melancholy; irritability.
5. Bronchitis; pleurisy; constant sneezing; tonsillitis; some coughs; madness; general body aches.
6. Sore throat; inability to speak; coughing; migraine; fever; pains in shoulders.
7. Migraine; toothaches; breathlessness; hemorrhoids; epilepsy; coughing; influenza; styes; shivering; excessive yawning; trembling; coldness in limbs.
8. Coughing; dry fever; heart pain; tonsillitis; pharyngitis; throat spasms.
9. Asthma; conjunctivitis; claustrophobia; excessive thirst; emphysema; nausea; vomiting; insomnia; heart pains.
10. Blood in mucus; vertigo; cholera; insomnia; excessive thirst; breast abscesses; coughing.

11. Meningitis; shivering; night sweats; swollen throat; dry mouth and lips; tonsillitis; fever; epilepsy.

SPLEEN
(*Figure 21: Leg Greater Yin Meridian*)

 1. Hemorrhoids; overacidity; madness; severe nausea; paralysis of feet.
 2. Lumbago; blurred vision; indigestion; difficulty in digesting food; swollen abdomen; heavy feeling in body.
 3. Heart pain; lumbago; constipation; intestinal pain; fever; anger.
 4. Pleurisy; internal hemorrhage; swollen abdomen; high fever.
 5. Sterility; nightmares; indigestion; hernia; stomach pain; great hunger but inability to digest food; jaundice.
 6. Insomnia; nervous depression; dysuria; genital pain; all diseases of sex organs in both men and women.
 7. Flatulence; inability to gain weight; indigestion; swollen ankles.
 8. Hemorrhoids; lumbago; irregular menstruation; fever.
 9. Body weakness; cramps; pain in joints; heaviness in abdomen.
10. Various intestinal disorders; eczema.
11. Gonorrhea; urinary problems.
12. Hernia; intestinal diseases; insufficient milk in mothers; swollen and painful lower abdomen.
13. Stomach pain; hernia; indigestion.
14. Coughing; constant perspiration; internal pains not localized.
15. Constipation; colitis; influenza; weakness in arms and legs.
16. Peptic ulcers; blood and pus in stool; under- or overacidity; internal hemorrhage.
17. Various general body aches, heaviness, and fever.
18. Peptic ulcers; swollen breasts; bronchitis; chest pain; coughing spells.
19. Bronchitis; lack of appetite; general aches.
20. Hemorrhoids; coughing; blood in sputum; eyes watery and swollen.
21. Pain and stiffness in various parts of body.

SMALL INTESTINE
(*Figure 22: Arm Greater Yang Meridian*)
 1. Convulsions in children; chest pains; heart pains; diarrhoea; polyuria.
 2. Epilepsy; sinus blockage; poor eyesight; neuralgia; dry fever; coryza.
 3. Stiff neck; tonsillitis; pruritus; epilepsy; madness; deafness; eye diseases; arm spasms.
 4. Pleurisy; eye diseases; vomiting; tinnitus; convulsions; meningitis; hemiplegia; headaches.
 5. Fainting; weakness; childhood fears; neuralgia in upper limbs; hemorrhoids; dizziness.
 6. Heaviness in arms; paralysis in arms; eyes red; vision dimmed.
 7. Excessive fear; vertigo; pain in hands; vertigo; swollen and painful throat.
 8. Insanity; shivering; tics; oedema of the heart; gingivitis.
 9. Numbness; neuritis; arthritis in arms; headache.
10. Arthritis; swelling in arms and legs.
11. Inability to move arms easily; facial swellings.
12. Pneumonia; pleurisy.
13. Inability to move arms easily; lack of coordination and strength in arms.
14. Pneumonia; muscle spasms in neck, shoulders, and arms.
15. Blood in mucus; weak eyesight; stiff neck; bronchitis.
16. Loss of coordination in upper half of body; muscle spasms in neck.
17. Nausea; vomiting; pleurisy; swollen tongue; neuralgia.
18. Toothache; inability to eat; stiffness in neck; numbness in face.
19. Deafness; hoarseness; sore throat; stiffness in jaw.

BLADDER
(*Figure 23: Leg Greater Yang Meridian*)
 1. All manner of eye diseases; headaches.
 2. Hallucinations; sinusitis; hay hever; watery eyes; blurred vision; nightmares; vomiting; redness and pain in eyes; eyes tire easily; stiff neck.
 3. Sinusitis; fainting; epilepsy; catarrh.
 4. Inability to perspire; facial neuralgia; nasal diseases.
 5. Heartburn; loss of memory; rigidity in spine; epilepsy; eye diseases.

6. Heart disease; visual problems; vomiting; palpitations; keratitis.
7. Chronic bronchitis; rhinitis; swelling and pain in face; excessive thirst and dryness in mouth.
8. Rheumatism; various emotional disorders; convulsions.
9. Continual weariness; myopia; vertigo; decreased vision; pains in eyes; neuralgia.
10. Nymphomania; lightheadedness; weakness in legs; nasal blockage; swollen throat; lack of body coordination.
11. Arthritis in lower joints; bronchitis; rheumatism; various bone diseases.
12. Sneezing fits; allergies; acne on body; asthma; coughing; dizziness accompanied by lightheadedness.
13. Pneumonia; asthma; coughing; gastritis; anorexia; lack of energy.
14. Sunstroke; heatstroke; heart pain; enlarged heart; pleurisy.
15. Emotional disorders; madness; vomiting; poor eyesight; flushed face; inability to stop talking.
16. Nervous breakdown; colic; flatulence; heart pain; stomach pains; alternating fever and chills.
17. Gastritis; pleurisy; night sweats; heart and chest pain.
18. Jaundice; asthma; duodenal ulcers; short temper; enlarged liver; bronchitis.
19. Weariness; pleurisy; high blood pressure; jaundice; yellow or bloodshot eyes.
20. Colitis; indigestion; gastritis; poor vision.
21. Inability to gain weight; internal hemorrhage; diarrhoea; gastritis; various stomach problems.
22. Urinary difficulties; stiffness in back and shoulder; inability to digest food.
23. Various kidney difficulties; excessive sexual dreams; asthma; weariness; premature ejaculation.
24. Gonorrhea; hemorrhoids.
25. Constipation; weakness in limbs; pain in lower abdomen.
26. Lumbago; diarrhoea; various bowel diseases.
27. Enteritis; colitis; blood in stool.
28. Leg and stomach pain; cystitis; dark urine; poor blood circulation.
29. Hernia; dysentery; kidney problems.
30. Paralysis in all four limbs; sciatica; urinary difficulties.

31. Impotence; constipation; inability to conceive; uterine prolapse; gonorrhea.
32. Genital diseases; sterility.
33. Genital diseases; diarrhoea; lower back pain; constipation; vomiting.
34. Genital diseases; lumbago; anuria.
35. Impotence; genital diseases; hemorrhoids; sciatica; gonorrhea.
36. Bronchitis; neuralgia.
37. Bronchitis; weakness in lungs.
38. Memory loss; anemia; severe weariness; emaciation
39. Asthma; various heart diseases.
40. Neuralgia; headache; fainting; poor vision; fever.
41. Various digestive disorders.
42. Rheumatism; pleurisy; difficulty in swallowing.
43. Rheumatism; flatulence; intestinal diseases that produce diarrhoea and vomiting.
44. Intestinal disorders; yellow in eyes; weariness; extreme thirst.
45. Backache; swollen abdomen; difficulty in swallowing.
46. Constipation; abdominal spasms; chest pains.
47. Weak kidneys; genital diseases.
48. Urethritis; gonorrhea; inflammation of testes.
49. Cystitis; various urinary diseases.
50. Sciatica; constipation; urinary difficulties; genital pain.
51. Poor circulation in lower limbs; bleeding hemorrhoids.
52. Cystitis; constipation; leg spasms; stiffness in legs.
53. Epilepsy; fainting; muscle spasms.
54. Skin diseases; loss of hair; nervousness; madness.
55. Hernia; various emotional disorders.
56. Constipation; muscle cramps; foot and leg pains.
57. Gonorrhea; epilepsy; loss of appetite and weight.
58. Cystitis; weakness; vertigo; epilepsy; lumbago; constipation; sciatica.
59. General body heaviness; inability to move limbs freely.
60. Diseases of the glands; vertigo; headache; childhood convulsions; poor eye control.
61. Gonorrhea; fainting; leg cramps; some emotional disorders.
62. Diseases of the spinal cord; headache due to tension; madness; dizziness; epilepsy.
63. General pain in lower abdomen; childhood convulsions.

64. Heart disease; madness; epilepsy; stiff neck; various cerebral disorders.
65. Abscesses; deafness; hemorrhoids.
66. Excessive fear; poor vision; gastritis; vertigo.
67. Genital diseases; fever; neuralgia; head and nose congestion; urinary difficulties.

LARGE INTESTINE
(*Figure 24: Arm Sunlight Yang Meridian*)

1. Swollen limbs; deafness; swollen neck; toothache; sudden colorblindness; laryngitis.
2. Toothache; jaundice; shivering; epistaxis; facial trembling.
3. Pain in eyes; tonsillitis; diarrhoea; neuralgia; swollen throat or tongue.
4. Bleeding gums; fever; tonsillitis; spots in front of eyes; migraine; deafness; paralysis in arms or legs; muteness; insomnia; depression.
5. Incoherence; dry fever; mucus cough; tonsillitis; uncontrollable laughter; tinnitus; toothache.
6. Fever; deafness; constipation; madness; tonsillitis.
7. Pain in arms; swollen throat or tongue; fever; madness.
8. Tuberculosis; weight loss; indigestion; blood in urine.
9. Gonorrhea; borborygmi; flatulence.
10. Pleurisy; muscle spasms in arms; poor circulation; tonsillitis; indigestion; pruritus; adenitis; toothaches.
11. Anemia; madness; epilepsy; pleurisy; swelling and pain in neck; redness in eyes.
12. Pain or numbness in arms and shoulders.
13. Pneumonia; blurred vision; peritonitis; melancholy; sleepiness; paralysis in arms and legs.
14. Stiff neck; fever; shivering; back pain.
15. High blood pressure; fever; muscle spasms; skin white and dry.
16. Toothache; epilepsy in children; emotional disorders.
17. Tonsillitis; throat diseases.
18. Sudden inability to speak; cough; shortness of breath.
19. Facial spasms; nasal problems; certain types of deafness.
20. Same as point 19, plus various facial disorders.

STOMACH
(*Figure 25: Leg Sunlight Yang Meridian*)

1. Deafness; night blindness; aversion to bright lights; spasms on face.

2. Dizziness; muteness; headache; watery eyes.
3. Nearsightedness; convulsions; paralysis of face; swollen feet.
4. Laryngitis; poor night vision; toothache; inability to speak.
5. Fever and chills; swollen glands; fits of madness.
6. Acne; glaucoma; laryngitis; spots in front of eyes.
7. Various visual difficulties; fainting; loose teeth.
8. Conjunctivitis; painful eyes; headache; facial numbness; aversion to bright lights; incessant blinking.
9. Sore and swollen throat; tonsillitis; vomiting.
10. Whooping cough; bronchitis; pruritus; tonsillitis.
11. Goiters; extreme excitability.
12. Nervous insomnia; cough; pleurisy; oedema; inability to stop talking.
13. Poor appetite; coughing; pleurisy; bronchitis.
14. Shock; blood in sputum; bronchitis; chest congestion.
15. Breast tumor; melancholy; itchiness; heaviness in arms; asthma; phlegm streaked with blood.
16. Emphysema; fever; heartburn; shortness of breath; ulcers on breast.
17. This point is not to be pierced—may result in insanity if used.
18. Hiccoughs; dry cough; long menstruation; chest pain.
19. Heart pain; cough; chest pain; indigestion; dryness in mouth.
20. Jaundice.
21. Upset stomach; gastritis; diarrhoea.
22. Bad breath; gastritis; swollen stomach; trembling accompanied by chills.
23. Madness; palpitations.
24. Vomiting; madness; rigid tongue.
25. Dysentery; fright; fatigue; bloated stomach; watery stool.
26. Pain in intestines.
27. Constipation; hernia; premature ejaculation; insomnia.
28. Nephritis; cystitis; diseased ovaries; rectal prolapse.
29. Sterility.
30. Impotence; hernia; stomach pain.
31. Gonorrhea; paralysis in limbs; muscle cramps.
32. Varicose veins; swollen abdomen; asthma at night.
33. Irregular menstruation; trembling hands; excessive thirst; hernia; paralysis.

34. Swollen breasts; cramps in stomach; numbness in arms or legs.
35. This point should not be pierced; may result in death.
36. Appendicitis; gastritis; indigestion; constipation; emaciation; nervousness; stomach pains; eye diseases.
37. Colitis; gastritis; diarrhoea; hemiplegia.
38. Rheumatism; tonsillitis; gastritis; diarrhoea.
39. Hair loss; inability to perspire; breast diseases.
40. Mental illness; asthma; muteness.
41. —Not used.
42. General feeling of coldness; desire to undress in public; aimless wandering; desire to climb on furniture; constant yawning; gingivitis; toothache.
43. High fever; swollen face; unusual thirst; coughing.
44. Toothache; gingivitis; diarrhoea; swollen abdomen.
45. Fitful sleep; sinusitis; fainting; rhinitis.

HEART
(*Figure 26: Arm Lesser Yin Meridian*)
1. Hysteria; depression; heart pain; low blood pressure; weak vision; impulsiveness; nausea; paralysis in arms and legs.
2. Fever; headache; spasms in arms; feeling of tightness across chest.
3. Depression; forgetfulness; chest pain; fainting; dizziness; epilepsy; madness; diseases of glands; nervous exhaustion.
4. Fear, anxiety; heart pain; hysteria; sudden inability to speak; nausea.
5. Many urinary diseases; palpitations; vertigo; headache; spasms in throat, neck, and arms; constipation; vomiting.
6. Shortness of breath; chest pain; chest congestion; fever alternating with chills; trembling in hands.
7. Hallucinations; constant sighing; heartbeat irregularities; incessant talking; forgetfulness; insomnia; fright; nasal inflammnation or blockage.
8. Uterine diseases; trembling; inability to urinate; hysteria; fear of people; fever.
9. Various heart diseases; irregularities in heartbeat and pulses; feeling of discouragement; pleurisy; difficulty in seeing clearly.

KIDNEYS
(*Figure 27: Leg Lesser Yin Meridian*)
 1. High blood pressure; measles; jaundice; vertigo; nasal bleeding; throat dry, painful, and tight; undue fear.
 2. Impotence; coughing up blood; dysentery; various genital diseases.
 3. Asthma; gonorrhea; migraine; undue sadness; insomnia; night madness; constipation; uterine prolapse.
 4. Impotence; myopia; menstrual difficulties.
 3. Asthma; gonorrhea; migraine; unduc sadness; insom-
 6. Impotence, dry fever; toothache; irregular menstruation; chest pains; dark urine.
 7. Dysentery; inability to sweat or constant perspiration; flatulence; paralysis of feet and lower legs; poor vision; fatigue.
 8. Dysentery; genital diseases.
 9. Problems in pregnancy; impulsive odd behavior.
10. Impotence; genital pain; stiffness in joints.
11. Genital pain; weakness in legs; urethritis; pain in eyes.
12. Cystitis; inability to urinate; frigidity; genital pain.
13. Impotence; pain in loins; various genital disorders.
14. Hernia; indigestion; pain in lower stomach.
15. Colitis; menstrual difficulties; general body weakness.
16. Jaundice; urethritis.
17. Mental impatience; wish to die; overacidity; jaundice; undue sadness or depression.
18. Sterility; sharp pains in stomach; dark urine; stiffness in neck and back; vomiting; inability to digest food.
19. Jaundice; asthma; numerous stomach disorders.
20. Gastritis; severe fright; inability to digest food; diarrhoea; duodenal ulcer; emphysema.
21. Amnesia; problems in pregnancy such as vomiting, lack of appetite, and severe pains in sides.
22. Breast abscesses; fullness in chest; nasal blockage.
23. Chest, head, and nasal congestion; breast tumors and ulcers.
24. Insomnia; pleurisy; bronchitis; emotional disorders.
25. Wish to die; incessant coughing and inability to breathe deeply; hearing difficulties.
26. Bad temper; easily irritated; coughing; bronchitis; stomach and chest spasms.
27. Irritability; asthma; nervousness; headache.

BIBLIOGRAPHY

Part I: Sources in Chinese

Chang Chun-mai and Ting Wen-chiang. *K'e hsueh yu jen-hseng kuan* (Science and Philosophy of Living). Shanghai, 1923.

Chang Hui-chen. *Li Shih-chen* (Li Shih-chen: Ancient China's Eminent Pharmacologist). Peking, 1955.

Chang Ping-lin. "Hsang-han-lun tan-lun pen t'i tz'u" (Interpretation of the text of the Hsang-han-lun), *China Monthly,* I:6 (February, 1924).

Chao Wen-ping, ed. *Collected Works on Acupuncture.* Rev. by Chang Ting-kuei. Shanghai, 1925.

Chao Yu-ching. "Hsin Chung-kuo te Chung-i yao chi-chi wu-chuang hsu-hsiang ts'ai neng tsou-hsiang k'e-hsueh-hua" (New China's traditional physicians must prepare themselves ideologically), *Peking Journal of Chinese Medicine,* I (June, 1952), 11-14.

————. *Chen-chiu ju-men* (Introduction to Acupuncture). Peking, 1964.

Ch'en Pang-hsien. *Chung-kuo i-hsueh hsih* (A Medical History of China). Shanghai, 1937.

Ch'en Wu-chiu. "Chung-yang Kuo-i-kuan hsuan-yen" (Manifesto of the Institute for Chinese Medicine), *Journal of the Medical Research Society of China,* II (1936), 104-109.

Cheng Tan-an. *Chung-kuo chen-chiu-huei* (Chinese Acupuncture and Moxabustion). Peking, 1959.

Chiang Hsao-yuan. "I-hsieh kuan-yu. . . . Chung-kuei mi-hsin" (Chinese Superstitions About Medicine), *Offerings,* II (August, 1928), 19-25.

Chiang Yu-po. *Chung-kuo yao-wu hsueh chi-ch'eng* (A Compendium of Chinese Pharmaceutical Products). Shanghai, 1935.

————. *Chung-i chin-hsiu tsu-chih kuan-li hsuan-chi* (Improving the Organization and Management of Chinese Medicine). Peking, 1953.

Huang Ti. *Huang Ti Nei-ching Su Wen* (The Yellow Emperor's Classic of Internal Medicine: Part I—Simple Questions). Peking, 1956.

Huang Ti. *Huang Ti Nei-Ching Ling Hsu* (The Yellow Emperor's Classic of Internal Medicine: Part II—The Mystic Gate [Nine Books]). Peking, 1927.

Hsieh Ti-yung, ed. *Chung-kuo i-yao fu-hsing hsih-lu* (The Medical Renaissance in China). Taipei, 1956.

Hsih Jo-lin. *Chung-kuo ku-tai te i-hsueh chiah* (The Physicians of Ancient China). Shanghai, 1958.

Su Yuan-chen, ed. *Chen-chiu pien-yung* (Acupuncture and Moxibustion Manual, with Prescriptions and Illustrations). Peking, 1903.

T'ien-min. "Chung-kuo tsui-ku fa-ming chih chen-chiu hsueh" (The Most Ancient Chinese Art of Acupuncture and Moxibustion), *Scientific China,* II (July, 1933), 4-5.

Yeh Ch'ing-chiu, ed. *Chung-i te hsueh-hsih tzu-liao* (Study Materials for Traditional Chinese Medicine). Shanghai, 1950.

BIBLIOGRAPHY

Part II: Sources in English and French

Baptiste, Roger. *L'Acupuncture et son histoire; Avantages et inconvenients d'une thérapeutique millénaire.* Paris: Librairie Maloine, 1962.

Berlioz, L.V.J. *Mémoires sur les maladies chroniques, les évacuations sanguine et l'acupuncture.* Paris: Chez Croullebois, 1816.

Bodde, Derek. *China's Cultural Tradition.* New York: Rinehart and Company, 1957.

Bourgeois, Gerard. *La Lutte contre le cancer par la physique nucléaire et l'acupuncture chinoise.* Paris: Editions Vega, 1950.

Buxton, L.H.D. *China: the Land and the People.* Oxford: Clarendon Press, 1929.

Chen, K.K. "Chinese Drug Stores," *Annals of Medical History,* VII (1925), 103-107.

———— and A.S.H. Ling. "Fragments of Chinese Medical History," *Annals of Medical History,* VIII (1926), 185-191.

Chen, Ronald. *The History and Methods of Physical Diagnosis in Classical Chinese Medicine.* New York: Vantage Press, 1969.

Ch'en, William Y. "Science in Communist China: Medicine and Public Health," *China Quarterly,* VI (April-June, 1961), 153-169.

Cowdry, E.V. "Medical Research in China," *Science,* LXII (1925), 374-377.

————. "Office of Imperial Physicians," *Journal of the American Medical Association,* LXXVII (1921), 307-312.

————. "Taoist Ideas of Anatomy," *Annals of Medical History,* III (1926), 301-309.

209

Croizier, Ralph C. *Traditional Medicine in Modern China.* Cambridge, Mass: Harvard University Press, 1968.

Dawson, P.M. "Su-Wen, the Basis of Chinese Medicine," *Annals of Medical History,* VII (1925), 59-67.

de la Fuye, Roger. *L'Acupuncture moderne pratique.* Paris: Le Francois, 1952.

————. *Traite d'acupuncture.* 2 vols. Paris: Le Francois, 1947.

De Lint, T.G. *Atlas of the History of Medicine.* New York: Paul B. Hoeber, Inc., 1920.

de Riencourt, Amaury. *The Soul of China: An Interpretation of Chinese History.* New York: Harper and Row, 1965.

Du Four, Roger. *Atlas d'acupuncture topographique.* Paris: Le Francois, 1960.

Edwards, E.D., ed. *The Dragon Book.* London: William Hodge and Co., Ltd., 1946.

Garrison, F.H. *Introduction to the History of Medicine.* Philadelphia: Saunders, 1929.

Giles, L. *The Sayings of Confucius.* London: Murray, 1907.

Glaser, Shirley. "Let Me Tell You About My Acupuncture," *New York Magazine,* IV (September 27, 1971), 64-65.

Goux, Henri. *Acupuncture.* Paris: Librairie Maloine, 1955.

Greene, Felix. *Awakened China.* Garden City, N.Y.: Doubleday, 1961.

Hashimoto, Masae. *Japanese Acupuncture.* Trans. by Keiko Suzuki. London: Thorsons, 1966.

Hellerman, Leon and Alan L. Stein, eds. *China: Readings on the Middle Kingdom.* New York: Simon & Schuster, 1971.

"Herb Medicine," *China Medical Journal,* LI (April, 1937), 552-553.

Horn, Joshua S. *Away With All Pests: An English Surgeon in People's China 1954-1969.* New York: Monthly Review Press, 1969.

Hsieh, E.T. "Notes from a Review of Ancient Chinese Anatomy," *Anatomical Record,* XX (1921), 97-127.

Huang Chia-ssu. "City Doctors Go to the Countryside," *China Reconstructs,* XIV (October, 1965), 30-33.

Huard, Pierre and Ming Wong. *Chinese Medicine.* Trans. by Bernard Fielding. New York: McGraw-Hill, 1968.

Hume, Edward Hicks. *The Chinese Way in Medicine.* Baltimore: The Johns Hopkins Press, 1940.

Kaltenmark, Odile. *Chinese Literature.* Trans. by Anne Marie Geoghegan. New York: Walker and Co., 1964.

Lavier, Jacques. *Histoire, doctrine et pratique de l'acupuncture chinoise.* Paris: Claude Tchou, Editeur, 1966.

————. *Points of Chinese Acupuncture.* Trans. by Dr. Phillip M. Chancellor. Rustington, Sussex, England: Health Science Press, 1965.

————. *Théorie et pratique de l'acupuncture.* Paris: Librairie Maloine, 1960.

Liang Yin. "Chinese Medicine Thrives on Modern and Traditional Methods," *Peking Review,* V (January 19, 1963), 15-17.

Liang Yung. "Integrating Chinese and Western Medicine," *Peking Review,* II (December 13, 1958), 21-23.

Lin Yutang, ed. *The Wisdom of China and India.* New York: Random House, 1942.

Loewe, Michael. *Everyday Life in Early Imperial China.* New York: G.P. Putnam's Sons, 1968.

Lu Wei-po and Yu Yung-ching. "Learning from Ancient China's Medicine," *China Reconstructs,* VIII (October, 1959), 32-34.

Lui, Garding. *Secrets of Chinese Physicians.* Los Angeles: B.N. Roberston Publishers, 1943.

Mann, Felix. *Acupuncture, the Ancient Chinese Art of Healing.* London: William Heinemann Medical Books, 1962.

————. *The Meridians of Acupuncture.* London: William Heinemann Medical Books, 1964.

————. *The Treatment of Disease by Acupuncture.* London: William Heinemann Medical Books, 1967.

Mi Ching-sen. "Ginseng, China's Famous Medicinal Root," *China Reconstructs,* XIII (May, 1964), 43-44.

Min Wang-chi. "China's Contribution to Medicine in the Past," *Annals of Medical History,* VIII (1926), 192-195.

Morgan, Edward. "Chinese Medicine," *West China Border Research Society Journal,* III (1926-1927), 116-142.

Morse, William B. *Chinese Medicine.* New York: Paul B. Hoeber (Clio Medica), 1934.

Moss, Louis. *Acupuncture and You.* New York: The Citadel Press, 1966.

Nakayama, T. *Acupuncture et médicine chinoise verifées au Japan.* Paris: Collection "Hippocrate," 1934.

Needham, Joseph and Lu Kuei-jen. "Hygiene and Preventive Medicine in Ancient China," *Journal of the History of Medicine and Allied Sciences,* XVII (October, 1962), 429-478.

Niboyet, J.E.H. *Complément d'acupuncture.* Paris: Wapler, 1955.

———. *Essai sur l'acupuncture chinoise pratique.* Paris: Wapler, 1951.

———. *Le Traitment d'algies par l'acupuncture.* Paris: Jacques Lafitte, 1959.

Orleans, Leo A. *Professional Manpower and Education in Communist China.* Washington, D.C., 1960.

Read, Bernard E. "Chinese Materia Medica," *China Medical Journal,* XXXVI (1922), 303-305 and XXXVIII (1924), 637-641.

———. "Chinese Materia Medica: A Review of Some of the Work of the Last Decade," *China Medical Journal,* LIV (April, 1938), 353-362.

———. "Chinese Pharmacopoeia," *China Medical Journal,* ILIV (June, 1930), 519-526.

———. "Gleanings from Old Chinese Medicine," *Annals of Medical History,* VIII (1926), 16-19.

Saar, John. "A Prickly Panacea Called Acupuncture," *Life,* LXXI (August 13, 1971), 32-35.

Sakurazawa, Yukikazu. *L'Acupuncture et la médicine d'Extrême-Orient.* Paris: J. Vrin, 1969.

The Science of Oriental Medicine: Its Principles and Methods. Los Angeles: The Foo and Wing Herb Co., Inc., 1902.

Stevenson, William. *The Yellow Wind.* Boston: Houghton Mifflin Co., 1959.

Stiefvater, Erich W. *What is Acupuncture? How Does it Work?* Rustington, Sussex, England: Health Science Press, 1962.

T'ang Yung-t'ung. "Wang Pi's New Interpretation of the I Ching and Lun-yu," trans. by Walter Liebenthal, *Harvard Journal of Asiatic Studies,* X (1947), 124-161.

Veith, Ilza. "Acupuncture Therapy—Past and Present," *Journal of the American Medical Association,* CLXXX (May 12, 1962), 478-484.

———. *The Yellow Emperor's Classic of Internal Medicine.* Berkeley and Los Angeles: University of California Press, 1966 (c. 1949).

Waley, Arthur. *Three Ways of Thought in Ancient China.* London: Allen and Unwin, 1939.

Wallnofer, Heinrich and Anna von Rottauscher. *Chinese*

Folk Medicine. New York: Bell Publishing Co., 1965.

Wang Chi-min. "China's Contribution to Medicine in the Past," *Annals of Medical History,* VIII (1926), 192-201.

Werner, E.T. *Myths and Legends of China.* London: Harrup, 1922.

Wilhelm, Richard and Cary F. Baynes, trans. *The I Ching or Book of Changes.* Princeton: The Princeton University Press, 1950.

Wing Tsit-chan, ed. and trans. *A Source Book in Chinese Philosophy.* Princeton: The Princeton University Press, 1963.

Wong, K.C. "China's Contribution to the Science of Medicine," *China Medical Journal,* ILIII (1929), 1193-1194.

———. and L.T. Wu. *History of Chinese Medicine.* Tientsin: Tientsin Press, n.d.

Woolley, Sir Leonard. *The Beginnings of Civilization.* New York: New American Library, 1965.

Wright, Arthur, ed. *Studies in Chinese Thought.* Chicago: University of Chicago Press, 1953.

Wu, S.C. "Chinese Medicine," *Chinese Recorder: Journal of the Christian Movement in China,* LVI (November, 1925), 733-741.

Wu Wei-ping. *Formulaire d'acupuncture.* Paris: Librairie Maloine, 1959.

Ying, King (Mrs. Yulin Hsi). *Chinese Medical Science in Practice.* Kowloon, Hong Kong, 1964.

Yueh Sung-sheng. "A Traditional Medicine Shop," *China Reconstructs,* XI (March, 1962), 41-43.

Index

(Page numbers italicized indicate illustration)

215

intestine, small, 64, 66, *74*; meridian of, *95*, 102, *105*, *119*, 130; pulse of, 145
In the Depth of the Pillow, 48
I Tsung, Emperor, 32-33
Ivy, Dr. Andrew, 26

jaundice, 122
Jen Min Chih Bao, 21-22
Jen Tsung, Emperor, 88
Jou to k'ou (nutmeg), 177
Ju hsiang (pistachio), 178
Juliana, Queen of the Netherlands, 11

Kan ts'ao (licorice), 178
Kao Ti, Emperor, 52
Kepler, Johannes, 49
kidney ailments, 178
kidneys, 64, 66, 67, *73*, 78, 87, 92; meridian of, *95*, 102, *110*, *125*, 131; pulse of, 145
Kim Bong-han, Professor, 21
Ko Huan, 47
Ko Hung (Pao P'u-tzu), 47-48, 49
Korea, acupuncture research in, 21-22
Krebiozen, 26
Kuan Yun Chang, 34
Kuomintang, 57, 58-59, 83

Lan Ong, 43
Lao Tzu, 46
laryngitis, 22, 122
laxatives, 178
L-Dopa drug, 21
Leg Absolute Yin (liver) meridian, 95, *95*, *97*, *112*, 131
Leg Greater Yang (bladder) meridian, *95*, 102, *106*, *120*, 131
Leg Greater Yin (spleen) meridian, *95*, 102, *104*, *117*, 130

Leg Lesser Yang (gallbladder), meridian, *95*, *99*, 100, *115*, 131
Leg Lesser Yin (kidney) meridian, *95*, 102, *110*, *125*, 131
Leg Sunlight Yang (stomach) meridian, *95*, 102, *108*, *123*, 130
leprosy, 47, 79, 87
Lian ch'ao (weeping forsythia), 177
Lien tzu (lotus flower), 177
Life magazine, 24-25
Ling Ti, Emperor, 42
Liou, Tsiang-lu, 44
Li Shih-chen, Dr., 52-53
listlessness, 173
liver, 64, 65-66, *71*, 77-78, 95, 100-101; meridian of, *95*, *97*, *112*, 131; pulse of, 145
Lon Nol, Premier of Cambodia, 11, 25
lumbago, 22, 45, 122
lung congestion, 45
lungs, 64, 65, 66, 67, *73*, 78, 126; meridian of, *95*, 102, *103*, *116*; pulse of, 145
Luo channels, 118
lymphangitis, acute, 47
lymphatic system, 69

Ma huang (Chinese ephedra), 178
malaria, 2, 59-60, 178
Mann, Felix, 23
Mao Tse-tung, 6, 7, 8, 13, 16, 58, 61-62, 181
Marx, Karl, 62
Massachusetts Institute of Technology, 5
massage, Chinese, 1, 92, 178-79
Mauries, Dr. J., 22-23
measles, 87
meningism, 122
menopause, rheumatism after, 22
menstrual difficulties, 22, 126